Dosage Calculations

made Incredibly Easy!

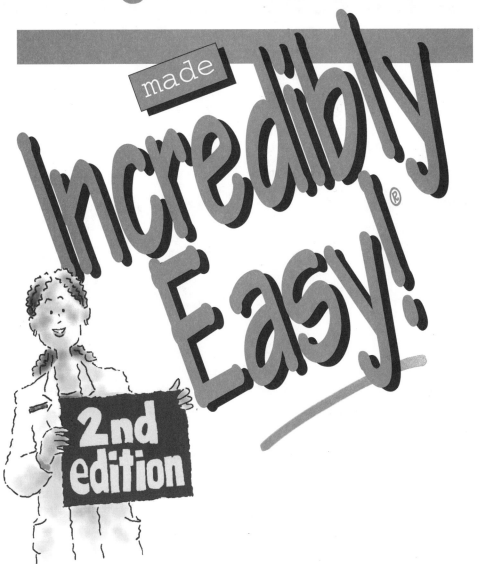

2nd edition

Springhouse
Springhouse, Pennsylvania

Staff

Publisher
Judith A. Schilling McCann, RN, MSN

Executive Editor
Kate Jackson

Clinical Manager
Joan M. Robinson, RN, MSN, CCRN

Clinical Editors
Collette Bishop Hendler, RN, CCRN
(clinical project manager);
Pamela Kovach, RN, BSN

Editors
Brenna H. Mayer (senior associate editor),
Cheryl L. Duksta, Ty Eggenberger,
Stacey Ann Follin, Kevin Haworth,
Kirk Robinson

Copy Editors
Jaime L. Stockslager (supervisor),
Kimberly Bilotta, Tom DeZego,
Heather Ditch, Mary T. Durkin,
Carolyn Petersen, Dorothy P. Terry,
Pamela Wingrod

Designers
Arlene Putterman (associate design
director), Mary Ludwicki (art director),
Lynn Foulk

Illustrators
Jackie Facciolo, Bot Roda

Electronic Production Services
Diane Paluba (manager), Joyce Rossi Biletz

Manufacturing
Patricia K. Dorshaw (manager),
Otto Mezei (book production manager)

Projects Coordinator
Liz Schaeffer

Editorial Assistants
Beverly Lane, Beth Janae Orr,
Elfriede Young

Indexer
Barbara Hodgson

Library of Congress Cataloging-in-Publication Data

Dosage calculation made incredibly easy.—2nd ed.
    p. ; cm.
    Includes index.
    1. Pharmaceutical arithmetic. I. Springhouse
Corporation.
    [DNLM: 1. Pharmaceutical Preparations—ad-
ministration & dosage—Nurses' instruction.
2. Mathematics—Nurses' Instruction.
QV 748 D722 2001]
RS57 .D67 2001
615′. 14—dc21
ISBN 1-58255-134-0 (alk. paper)   2001020924

Contents

Contributors and consultants iv

Foreword v

Part I   Math basics

1 Fractions 3
2 Decimals and percentages 25
3 Ratios, fractions, proportions, and solving for X 45
4 Dimensional analysis 65

Part II   Measurement systems

5 Metric system 77
6 Alternative measurement systems 91

Part III   Recording drug administration

7 Drug orders 109
8 Administration records 121

Part IV   Oral, topical, and rectal drugs

9 Calculating oral drug dosages 135
10 Calculating topical and rectal drug dosages 163

Part V   Parenteral administration

11 Calculating parenteral injections 175
12 Calculating I.V. infusions 205

Part VI   Special calculations

13 Calculating pediatric dosages 235
14 Calculating obstetric drug dosages 255
15 Calculating critical care dosages 269

Appendices and index

Practice makes perfect 284
Glossary 302
Index 305

Contributors and consultants

Margaret M. Gingrich, RN, MSN
Associate Professor
Harrisburg (Pa.) Area Community College

Rebecca Crews Gruener, RN, MS
Associate Professor of Nursing
Louisiana State University at Alexandria

Dr. Joyce Lyne Heise, EdD
Associate Professor of Nursing
Kent State University
East Liverpool, Ohio

Erin Jaynes, RN, MSN
Associate Professor of Nursing
Owens Community College
Toledo, Ohio

Holly K. Kailani, RN,C, MSN
Assistant Professor of Nursing
Hawaii Pacific University
Kaneohe

Dr. Patricia A. Lange-Otsuka, RN, EdD, APRN, CCRN
Associate Professor of Nursing
Graduate Nursing Program Coordinator
Hawaii Pacific University
Kaneohe

Samir Ouzomgi, PhD
Associate Professor of Mathematics
Pennsylvania State University
Abington

Sylvia Ouzomgi, RN, MPA, CCRN
Nursing Supervisor
Montgomery Hospital
Norristown, Pa.

Patricia Harvey Webb, RN,C, EdD
Associate Professor of Nursing
Samuel Merritt College, School of Nursing
Oakland, Calif.

Joyce Welliver, RN, MSN, CRNP
Assistant Professor
Holy Family College
Philadelphia

Rosemarie C. Westberg, RN, MSN, CPN
Professor of Nursing
Northern Virginia Community College
Annandale

We extend special thanks to the following people who contributed to the previous edition:

Lillian S. Brunner, RN, MSN, FAAN, DSC
Bridget A. Haupt, PharmD
Catherine Nebe, RPh
Margaret R. Rateau, RN, MSN
Nancy V. Runta, RN,C, MSN, CCRN
Maryann Summers, RN, MS
David L. Wolff
Bonnie Zauderer, RN, MS, CNS

Foreword

In this era of the unit-dose system, some health care professionals believe that they've been absolved of their responsibility for accurately determining drug calculations. However, safe practice demands that calculations be made correctly to ensure that medications are administered accurately. Dosage calculation requires not only proficiency in math but also critical thinking about the process and the product of the calculation. Patients' well-being — and even their lives — may depend on these calculations and critical thinking skills. Furthermore, the ability to accurately determine the dose of a drug is a responsibility for which all nurses are held legally accountable.

Unfortunately, many practicing nurses and students believe that, when it comes to math, they're doomed to failure. That's why the clinical experts at Springhouse have created the second edition of *Dosage Calculations Made Incredibly Easy*. This book challenges the notion that mastery of math is beyond our reach. Students, practicing nurses, and inactive nurses planning to return to the work force — professionals responsible for drug administration — can benefit from this fantastic book. It's suitable for individual study, small group sessions, or classroom discussions.

This book isn't like any other dosage calculation book you've read. The straightforward approach, which includes a variety of learning techniques and abundant humor, makes *Dosage Calculations Made Incredibly Easy*, Second Edition, fun, practical, and informative. The concise, step-by-step format makes learning easy and enjoyable.

The first section of the book helps you master the basics. After fractions are thoroughly explained, concepts associated with decimals and percentages are discussed and illustrated and the rules for ratios, fractions, proportions, and solving for X are made clear. This section contains details about working with different types of fractions; converting fractions; adding, subtracting, multiplying, and dividing fractions and decimal fractions; and solving percentage problems, decimal-fraction equations, and proportion problems with ratios and fractions. A new chapter on dimensional analysis introduces the popular method for systematically converting units on the drug package to units on the order. Numerous definitions, examples, and illustrations make mastery easy.

Conversions between the various measurement systems are followed by information on drug orders, avoiding drug errors, and documenting medication administration. Helpful advice on military time, standard abbreviations, dealing with unclear drug orders, computerized patient records, recording drug information, and ensuring quality care make *Dosage Calculations Made Incredibly Easy*, Second Edition, more than a math book.

Each chapter begins with learning objectives and ends with a quiz so you can determine if you achieved the chapter objectives. Throughout the book, sidebars summarize key points, and numerous illustrations clearly display examples of the topics discussed.

In the second edition, all information has been updated. The second edition also has a *Practice makes perfect* test with real-to-life case studies at the end of the book that allows you to bring all the concepts together to find which areas you've mastered and which need review.

Throughout the book, special logos alert you to important points:

Real world problems relates particular math concepts to practice situations you're likely to encounter in the work world.

For math phobics only provides additional explanations, illustrations, and examples of a given calculation problem so that even the most math-phobic student can understand the concept.

Advice from the experts keeps you on track and helps you remember the information you're learning.

Before you give that drug alerts you to information essential to avoiding medication administration errors.

Peak technique contains additional strategies to help you calculate and administer drugs accurately and safely.

Your role as a successful health care practitioner requires dosage calculation skills. And, let's face facts: Medication errors are unacceptable and can be dangerous to your patient's health. As you overcome the obstacles to developing math skills, you gain confidence in your ability to calculate drug dosages and administer medications accurately and safely. With its unique, entertaining approach, *Dosage Calculations Made Incredibly Easy*, Second Edition, will have you jumping over math hurdles like a pro. Happy calculating!

Veta H. Massey, RN, PhD
Dean, Division of Nursing
Baptist Memorial College of Health Sciences
Memphis

Part I

Math basics

1 **Fractions** 3

2 **Decimals and percentages** 25

3 **Ratios, fractions, proportions, and solving for** *X* 45

4 **Dimensional analysis** 65

① Fractions

Just the facts

In this chapter, you'll learn:

♦ what a fraction is

♦ about different types of fractions you may use

♦ how to convert fractions, reduce them to their lowest terms, and find the lowest common denominator

♦ how to add, subtract, multiply, and divide fractions.

A look at fractions

A fraction represents the division of one number by another number. It's a mathematical expression for parts of a whole. (See *Parts of a whole.*)

Parts of a whole

In any fraction, the numerator (top number) and the denominator (bottom number) represent the parts of the whole. The denominator describes the total number of equal parts in the whole; the numerator describes the number of parts being considered.

> The numerator is on the top.

> The denominator is on the bottom.

> The numerator 5 over the denominator 16 shows that we're considering 5 parts out of 16.

Getting to the bottom of it

The bottom number, or denominator, represents the total number of equal parts in the whole. The larger the denominator, the greater the number of equal parts. For example, in the fraction $\frac{3}{5}$, the denominator 5 indicates that the whole has been divided into five equal parts. In the fraction $\frac{7}{12}$, the denominator 12 indicates that the whole has been divided into 12 equal parts. So, as the denominator becomes larger, the size of the parts becomes smaller.

Staying on top of it

The top number, or numerator, signifies the number of parts of the whole being considered. For example, in the fraction $\frac{3}{5}$, only 3 of the 5 equal parts are being considered. In the fraction $\frac{7}{12}$, only 7 of the 12 equal parts are being considered.

Types of fractions

There are four types of fractions:
- common
- complex
- proper
- improper.

Common and complex

In a common fraction, such as $\frac{2}{3}$, both the numerator and denominator are whole numbers.

In a complex fractionthe numerator and denominator are fractions. For example:

$$\frac{2/7}{5/16}$$

Proper and improper

In a proper fraction, such as $\frac{1}{4}$, the numerator is smaller than the denominator.

In an improper fraction, such as $\frac{8}{7}$ or $11\frac{1}{4}$, the numerator is larger than the denominator. In other words, it's top heavy. An improper fraction represents a number that's greater than 1.

An improper fraction can also be expressed as a mixed number — a whole number and a fraction. Therefore, $\frac{8}{7}$ can be rewritten as $1\frac{1}{7}$ and $11\frac{1}{4}$ can be rewritten as $2\frac{3}{4}$.

Working with fractions

Cheat sheet

You can manipulate fractions in three ways, including:
• converting mixed numbers to improper fractions and vice versa
• reducing fractions to their lowest terms
• finding a common denominator.

Converting mixed numbers to improper fractions

To convert a mixed number to an improper fraction, follow these steps:

 Multiply the denominator by the whole number.

 Add the product, or resulting number, from the first step to the numerator (this gives you a new numerator).

 Leave the denominator as it is.

Three incredibly easy steps

For example, to convert the mixed number 5⅓ to an improper fraction:

 Multiply the denominator 3 by the whole number 5, for a total of 15.

 Add 15 to the numerator 1, for a new numerator of 16.

 Leave the denominator as it is. The improper fraction is ¹⁶⁄₃.

$$5\tfrac{1}{3} \text{ is } \frac{16}{3}$$

Encore!

Here's another another example! To convert the mixed number 8⅘ to an improper fraction:

 Multiply the denominator 5 by the whole number 8, for a total of 40.

 Add 40 to the numerator 4, for a new numerator of 44.

Making fractions work

Mixed numbers to improper fractions
• Multiply the denominator by the whole number.
• Add product to the numerator.
• Resulting sum is the new numerator.
• Leave the denominator as it is.

Reducing fractions
• Determine the largest common divisor.
• Divide both the numerator and denominator by that number.

Common denominators
• To find, multiply all the denominators in a set of fractions.
• The smallest multiple of the denominators is the lowest common denominator.

Leave the denominator as it is. The improper fraction is ⁴⁴⁄₅.

$$8\tfrac{4}{5} \text{ is } \frac{44}{5}$$

Putting it in reverse

At times, you may want to convert improper fractions back to mixed numbers. To convert the improper fraction ¹⁶⁄₃ back to a mixed number:

Divide the numerator 16 by the denominator 3. When you do this, you get 5 with 1 left over.

The 1 becomes the new numerator, and the denominator stays the same.

The mixed number is 5⅓:

$$\frac{16}{3} \text{ is } 5\tfrac{1}{3}$$

One more time

To convert the improper fraction ⁴⁴⁄₅ back into a mixed number:

Divide the numerator 44 by the denominator 5. The answer is 8 with 4 left over.

Place the 4 over the 5.

The mixed number is 8⅘.

$$\frac{44}{5} \text{ is } 8\tfrac{4}{5}$$

Reducing fractions to lowest terms

For simplicity's sake, a fraction should usually be reduced to its lowest terms — that is, to the smallest numbers possible in the numerator and denominator. To simplify a fraction, follow these steps:

✌ Determine the largest common divisor of the numerator and the denominator — the largest number by which both can be divided equally.

✌ Divide both the numerator and denominator by that number to reduce the fraction to its lowest terms.

Example numero uno

To reduce the fraction ⁸⁄₁₀ to its lowest terms:

✌ Determine the largest common divisor of 8 and 10, which is 2.

✌ Divide the numerator and denominator by 2 to reduce the fraction to its lowest terms, or ⅘.

$$\frac{8}{10} \text{ is } \frac{8 \div 2}{10 \div 2} \text{ is } \frac{4}{5}$$

Missed it? Watch again

To reduce the fraction ⁷⁄₁₄ to its lowest terms:

✌ Determine that the number 7 is the largest divisor that 7 and 14 have in common.

✌ Divide the numerator and the denominator by 7 to reduce the fraction to its lowest terms, or ½. This fraction can't be reduced further.

$$\frac{7}{14} \text{ is } \frac{7 \div 7}{14 \div 7} \text{ is } \frac{1}{2}$$

One more time

To reduce the fraction ²⁄₁₀ to its lowest terms:

✌ Determine that the number 2 is the largest divisor that 2 and 10 have in common.

✌ Divide the numerator and the denominator by 2 to reduce the fraction to its lowest terms, or ⅕.

$$\frac{2}{10} \text{ is } \frac{2 \div 2}{10 \div 2} \text{ is } \frac{1}{5}$$

Reducing a fraction to its lowest terms will make my life simpler!

Finding a common denominator

One way to find a common denominator for a set of fractions is to multiply all the denominators. For example, to find a common denominator for the fractions ⅖ and ⁷⁄₁₀, multiply the denominators 5 and 10 to get the multiplied common denominator 50:

Multiply the denominators...

$$\frac{2}{5} \quad \frac{7}{10}$$

...to find the multiplied common denominator.

$$5 \times 10 = 50$$

To find the multiplied common denominator of the set of fractions ⅛, ¼, and ⅕, simply multiply all the denominators together to find the common denominator 160:

$$8 \times 4 \times 5 = 160$$

Lowest common denominator

Unfortunately, multiplying all the denominators of a set of fractions won't always give you the lowest common denominator. The *lowest common denominator* or *least common multiple* — the smallest number that's a multiple of all the denominators in a set of fractions — is an important tool for working with fractions.

How low can you go?

One way to find the lowest common denominator of a set of fractions is to work with its prime factors. A *prime number* is a number that's evenly divisible only by 1 and itself. Some prime numbers are 2, 3, 5, and 7. *Prime factors* are prime numbers that can be divided into some part of a mathematical expression, in this case, the denominators in a set of fractions.

Prime factoring

Let's say you want to find the lowest common denominator for ⅛, ¼, and ⅕. Here's a useful technique, called *prime factoring:*
• Make a table with two headings: "Prime factors" and "Denominators."
• Write the denominators 8, 4, and 5 over the top right columns.

Prime factors	Denominators		
	8	4	5

• Divide the three denominators by the prime factors for each, starting with the smallest prime factor by which one of the denominators can be divided — in this case, 2. Write 2 in the left-hand column and divide the denominators by it. (Divide the denominator 8 by the prime factor 2 and write the answer, 4, in the column under the 8. Then divide the denominator 4 by the prime factor 2 and write the answer, 2, in the column under the denominator 4.)

• Bring down the numbers in the right-side columns that aren't evenly divisible by the prime factor in the left column. (In this case, the denominator 5 isn't divisible by the prime factor 2, so just bring the 5 down.)

Prime factors	Denominators		
2	8	4	5
	4	2	5

• Repeat this process until the numbers in the bottom row can't be divided further.

Prime factors	Denominators		
	8	4	5
2	4	2	5
2	2	1	5
2	1	1	5

• Then multiply the prime factors in the left column by the numbers in the bottom row. To say it with numbers:

$$2 \times 2 \times 2 \times 1 \times 1 \times 5 = 40$$

• The lowest common denominator for this set of fractions is 40.

Wow! Can you show me again?

OK. Let's use prime factoring to find the lowest common denominator for ⅜ and ⅚. Create a table that lists the denominators horizontally; then find the prime factors.

Here's what the table looks like:

Prime factors	Denominators		
	8	6	
2	4	3	
2	2	3	
2	1	3	

• Then multiply the prime factors in the left column by the numbers in the bottom row:

$$2 \times 2 \times 2 \times 1 \times 3 = 24$$

> Lowest common denominator

Once more, please

Now, use prime factoring to find the lowest common denominator for ⅓, ¼, and ½.

Here's the table:

Prime factors	Denominator		
	3	4	2
2	3	2	1
2	3	1	1

Then multiply the prime factors in the left column by the numbers in the bottom row:

$$2 \times 2 \times 3 \times 1 \times 1 = 12$$

> Lowest common denominator

Converting fractions

Once you know the lowest common denominator of a set of fractions, you can *convert* the fractions so that all have the same denominator — the *lowest common denominator*.

One way to convert a set of fractions is to multiply each fraction by 1 in the form of a fraction — that is, a fraction with the same number in the numerator and denominator. You can find this fraction by taking the lowest common denominator and dividing it by the original denominator.

Here's what the formula looks like:

$$\frac{\text{original}}{\text{fraction}} \times \frac{\text{lowest common denominator} \div \text{original denominator}}{\text{lowest common denominator} \div \text{original denominator}}$$

> This is how you convert a fraction using 1 in the form of a fraction.

Conversion excursion

Convert the set of fractions ⅛, ¼, and ⅕ so that each has the lowest common denominator. We already know that the lowest common denominator for this set of fractions is 40.

- Here's the conversion of the first fraction, ⅛, to ⁵⁄₄₀:

$$\frac{1}{8} = \frac{1}{8} \times \frac{40 \div 8}{40 \div 8} = \frac{1}{8} \times \frac{5}{5} = \frac{1 \times 5}{8 \times 5} = \frac{5}{40}$$

- Convert the next fraction, ¼, to ¹⁰⁄₄₀:

$$\frac{1}{4} = \frac{1}{4} \times \frac{40 \div 4}{40 \div 4} = \frac{1}{4} \times \frac{10}{10} = \frac{1 \times 10}{4 \times 10} = \frac{10}{40}$$

- Convert the last fraction in the set, ⅕, to ⁸⁄₄₀:

$$\frac{1}{5} = \frac{1}{5} \times \frac{40 \div 5}{40 \div 5} = \frac{1}{5} \times \frac{8}{8} = \frac{1 \times 8}{5 \times 8} = \frac{8}{40}$$

Do it again

This is how to convert ⅜ and ⅚ to fractions with the lowest common denominator, which is 24.

- Convert the first fraction, ⅜, to ⁹⁄₂₄:

$$\frac{3}{8} = \frac{3}{8} \times \frac{24 \div 8}{24 \div 8} = \frac{3}{8} \times \frac{3}{3} = \frac{3 \times 3}{8 \times 3} = \frac{9}{24}$$

- Convert the other fraction, ⅚, to ²⁰⁄₂₄:

$$\frac{5}{6} = \frac{5}{6} \times \frac{24 \div 6}{24 \div 6} = \frac{5}{6} \times \frac{4}{4} = \frac{5 \times 4}{6 \times 4} = \frac{20}{24}$$

Once more

OK. Now convert ⅓, ¼, and ½ to fractions with the lowest common denominator, which is 12.

- Convert ⅓ to ⁴⁄₁₂:

$$\frac{1}{3} = \frac{1}{3} \times \frac{12 \div 3}{12 \div 3} = \frac{1}{3} \times \frac{4}{4} = \frac{1 \times 4}{3 \times 4} = \frac{4}{12}$$

- Convert ¼ to ³⁄12:

$$\frac{1}{4} = \frac{1}{4} \times \frac{12 \div 4}{12 \div 4} = \frac{1}{4} \times \frac{3}{3} = \frac{1 \times 3}{4 \times 3} = \frac{3}{12}$$

- Convert the last fraction, ½, to ⁶⁄12:

$$\frac{1}{2} = \frac{1}{2} \times \frac{12 \div 2}{12 \div 2} = \frac{1}{2} \times \frac{6}{6} = \frac{1 \times 6}{2 \times 6} = \frac{6}{12}$$

Divide and conquer

You can also convert a set of fractions by using long division. To convert each fraction, follow these steps:

☝   Divide the lowest common denominator by the original denominator.

✌   Multiply the quotient, or resulting number, by the original numerator to determine the new numerator.

🖐   Place the new numerator over the lowest common denominator.

Here's how to set up the conversion for each fraction:

$$\overset{\displaystyle \text{quotient}}{\underset{\text{denominator}}{\text{original}}\overline{\big)\,\underset{\text{denominator}}{\text{lowest common}}}} \times \overset{\text{original}}{\underset{}{\text{numerator}}} = \frac{\text{new numerator}}{\underset{\text{denominator}}{\text{lowest common}}}$$

Set 'em up

This is how to convert ³⁄8, ¼, and ²⁄5. The lowest common denominator is 40.

- Convert the first fraction in the set, ³⁄8, to ¹⁵⁄40:

$$\frac{3}{8} = 8\overline{)40}^{\,5} \times 3 = \frac{15}{40}$$

- Convert ¼ to ¹⁰⁄40:

$$\frac{1}{4} = 4\overline{)40}^{\,10} \times 1 = \frac{10}{40}$$

- Convert ²⁄5 to ¹⁶⁄40:

$$\frac{2}{5} = 5\overline{)40}^{\,8} \times 2 = \frac{16}{40}$$

Amazing! Let's see that again

This is how to convert ⅜ and ⅚. The lowest common denominator is 24.

- Convert the fraction ⅜ to 9/24:

$$\frac{3}{8} = 8\overline{)24}^{\,3} \times 3 = \frac{9}{24}$$

- Convert ⅚ to 20/24:

$$\frac{5}{6} = 6\overline{)24}^{\,4} \times 5 = \frac{20}{24}$$

One last time

And this is how to convert ⅓, ¼, and ½. The lowest common denominator is 12.

- Convert ⅓ to 4/12:

$$\frac{1}{3} = 3\overline{)12}^{\,4} \times 1 = \frac{4}{12}$$

- Convert ¼ to 3/12:

$$\frac{1}{4} = 4\overline{)12}^{\,3} \times 1 = \frac{3}{12}$$

- Convert ½ to 6/12:

$$\frac{1}{2} = 2\overline{)12}^{\,6} \times 1 = \frac{6}{12}$$

I can convert this set of fractions!

Comparing fraction size

Why are these calculations important? Because finding the lowest common denominator in a set of fractions allows you to compare the relative size of the fractions. This concept is extremely useful for comparing the strengths of medications. (See *Denominators can be deceptive*, page 14.)

Oh, boy! A real world application

For example, suppose you want to compare the strengths of sublingual nitroglycerin tablets, which are available in 1/100-grain, 1/150-grain, and 1/200-grain strengths. Follow these steps:

The Real World

- Using the prime factor method, first find the lowest common denominator for these three fractions. The table looks like this:

Prime factors	Denominators		
	100	150	200
2	50	75	100
2	25	75	50
5	5	15	10
5	1	3	2

- Then multiply the prime factors in the left column and the numbers in the bottom row. In other words:

$$2 \times 2 \times 5 \times 5 \times 1 \times 3 \times 2 = 600$$

> Lowest common denominator

Finding common ground

Next, convert all three fractions — $\frac{1}{100}$, $\frac{1}{150}$, and $\frac{1}{200}$ — to new fractions with the lowest common denominator of 600. To do this, multiply each fraction by 1 in the form of a fraction (create this

For math phobics only

Denominators can be deceptive

If you were hungry, would you rather have 1 slice from a pie that was cut into 4 slices, 8 slices, or 16 slices? You'd choose 4, of course, because the slices would be bigger. You can judge the size of fractions the same way. When the fractions all have the same numerators — in this case, $\frac{1}{4}$, $\frac{1}{8}$, and $\frac{1}{16}$ — the fraction with the lowest denominator is the biggest one. Don't fall into the trap of thinking that the bigger the denominator, the bigger the fraction. Think in terms of a pie, as shown below.

fraction by dividing the lowest common denominator by the original denominator).

Here's the conversion:

- The fraction $\frac{1}{100}$ is converted to $\frac{6}{600}$:

$$\frac{1}{100} = \frac{1}{100} \times \frac{600 \div 100}{600 \div 100} = \frac{1}{100} \times \frac{6}{6} = \frac{1 \times 6}{100 \times 6} = \frac{6}{600}$$

- $\frac{1}{150}$ is converted to $\frac{4}{600}$:

$$\frac{1}{150} = \frac{1}{150} \times \frac{600 \div 150}{600 \div 150} = \frac{1}{150} \times \frac{4}{4} = \frac{1 \times 4}{150 \times 4} = \frac{4}{600}$$

- $\frac{1}{200}$ is converted to $\frac{3}{600}$:

$$\frac{1}{200} = \frac{1}{200} \times \frac{600 \div 200}{600 \div 200} = \frac{1}{200} \times \frac{3}{3} = \frac{1 \times 3}{200 \times 3} = \frac{3}{600}$$

Comparing the three final fractions, you'll see that the $\frac{1}{100}$-grain nitroglycerin tablet offers the largest dose: $\frac{6}{600}$.

Same destination, different route

You can arrive at the same conclusion by dividing the lowest common denominator (600) by the denominator, multiplying the numerator by the number obtained, and placing the result over the lowest common denominator.

- The fraction $\frac{1}{100}$ is converted to $\frac{6}{600}$ this way:

$$\frac{1}{100} = 100\overline{)600}^{\ 6} \times 1 = \frac{6}{600}$$

- $\frac{1}{150}$ is converted to $\frac{4}{600}$:

$$\frac{1}{150} = 150\overline{)600}^{\ 4} \times 1 = \frac{4}{600}$$

- $\frac{1}{200}$ is converted to $\frac{3}{600}$:

$$\frac{1}{200} = 200\overline{)600}^{\ 3} \times 1 = \frac{3}{600}$$

The lowest common denominator is the key.

Fraction fact

When comparing fractions with common denominators, the fraction with the largest numerator is the largest number. In the set of fractions above, $\frac{6}{600}$ is the largest number.

A common hero

The lowest common denominator also enables you to add and subtract fractions. Reducing fractions to their lowest terms and converting improper fractions to mixed numbers lets you present the answers to addition, subtraction, multiplication, and division problems in a useful way.

Remember: Whenever you perform these functions, always reduce the final answer to its lowest terms and, if it's an improper fraction, convert it to a mixed number.

Adding fractions

To add fractions, first convert them to fractions with common denominators. (See *Comparing apples to apples.*)

It all adds up

Here's an example of adding fractions. Follow the steps below to add the fractions ½ and ⅓.

Find the lowest common denominator. Because the denominators in ½ and ⅓ are both prime numbers, multiply 7 by 3 to find the lowest common denominator, 21.

Then convert the fractions by multiplying each by 1 (in the form of a fraction) to yield fractions with the lowest common denominator.

Start by converting ½ to ³⁄₂₁:

$$\frac{1}{7} = \frac{1}{7} \times \frac{21 \div 7}{21 \div 7} = \frac{1}{7} \times \frac{3}{3} = \frac{1 \times 3}{7 \times 3} = \frac{3}{21}$$

Then convert ⅓ to ⁷⁄₂₁:

$$\frac{1}{3} = \frac{1}{3} \times \frac{21 \div 3}{21 \div 3} = \frac{1}{3} \times \frac{7}{7} = \frac{1 \times 7}{3 \times 7} = \frac{7}{21}$$

Now, add the new fractions. To add fractions with a common denominator, add the numerators and place the result over the common denominator. The resulting fraction is your answer. (Reduce it to its lowest terms, if possible.)

$$\frac{3}{21} + \frac{7}{21} = \frac{3 + 7}{21} = \frac{10}{21}$$

SNAP

Additional addition

To add ½ and ⅕, follow these steps.

Comparing apples to apples

When adding or subtracting fractions, don't forget to convert them to fractions with common denominators. That way, you'll be comparing apples to apples.

 Find the lowest common denominator. In this case, because the denominators 2 and 5 are both prime numbers, multiply 2 by 5 to find the lowest common denominator, 10.

Convert the fractions by multiplying each by 1 (in the form of a fraction) to yield fractions with the lowest common denominator.

 Convert the fraction ½ to ⁵⁄₁₀:

$$\frac{1}{2} = \frac{1}{2} \times \frac{10 \div 2}{10 \div 2} = \frac{1}{2} \times \frac{5}{5} = \frac{1 \times 5}{2 \times 5} = \frac{5}{10}$$

Then convert ⅕ to ²⁄₁₀:

$$\frac{1}{5} = \frac{1}{5} \times \frac{10 \div 5}{10 \div 5} = \frac{1}{5} \times \frac{2}{2} = \frac{1 \times 2}{5 \times 2} = \frac{2}{10}$$

Now, add the converted fractions. To do this, add the numerators and place the result over the common denominator:

$$\frac{5}{10} + \frac{2}{10} = \frac{5 + 2}{10} = \frac{7}{10}$$

Another additional addition

To add ⅗ and ⅔, follow these steps.

 Find the lowest common denominator — in this case, 15.

Convert the fractions by multiplying each by 1 (in the form of a fraction) to yield fractions with the lowest common denominator.

Convert ⅗ to 9/15:

$$\frac{3}{5} = \frac{3}{5} \times \frac{15 \div 5}{15 \div 5} = \frac{3}{5} \times \frac{3}{3} = \frac{3 \times 3}{5 \times 3} = \frac{9}{15}$$

Then convert ⅔ to ¹⁰/15:

$$\frac{2}{3} = \frac{2}{3} \times \frac{15 \div 3}{15 \div 3} = \frac{2}{3} \times \frac{5}{5} = \frac{2 \times 5}{3 \times 5} = \frac{10}{15}$$

To add the converted fractions, add the new numerators and place the result over the common denominator:

$$\frac{9}{15} + \frac{10}{15} = \frac{9 + 10}{15} = \frac{19}{15}$$

Reduce the fraction to its lowest terms:

$$\frac{19}{15} = 1\frac{4}{15}$$

It all adds up!

Subtracting fractions

Like addition, subtraction requires converting fractions to terms with common denominators.

Fraction subtraction

Here's an example of how to subtract one fraction from another. Follow the steps below to subtract ⅙ from 5/12.

Find the lowest common denominator — in this case, 12. The fraction 5/12 already has the lowest common denominator.

Convert the fraction ⅙ to a fraction with the lowest common denominator. To do this, multiply the fraction by the number 1 (in the form of a fraction).

$$\frac{1}{6} = \frac{1}{6} \times \frac{12 \div 6}{12 \div 6} = \frac{1}{6} \times \frac{2}{2} = \frac{1 \times 2}{6 \times 2} = \frac{2}{12}$$

Now, subtract the numerators and place the result over the common denominator:

$$\frac{5}{12} - \frac{2}{12} = \frac{5 - 2}{12} = \frac{3}{12}$$

Reduce the fraction to its lowest terms, if possible. The resulting fraction is your answer:

$$\frac{3}{12} = \frac{1}{4}$$

A second subtraction

To subtract ⅑ from ⅚, follow these steps.

Find the lowest common denominator—in this case, 18. (To find the lowest common denominator in this case, try prime factoring on your own.)

Convert the fractions to those with the lowest common denominator by multiplying each fraction by the number 1 (in the form of a fraction).

Convert ⅚ to ¹⁵⁄₁₈:

$$\frac{5}{6} = \frac{5}{6} \times \frac{18 \div 6}{18 \div 6} = \frac{5}{6} \times \frac{3}{3} = \frac{5 \times 3}{6 \times 3} = \frac{15}{18}$$

Then convert ⅑ to ²⁄₁₈:

$$\frac{1}{9} = \frac{1}{9} \times \frac{18 \div 9}{18 \div 9} = \frac{1}{9} \times \frac{2}{2} = \frac{1 \times 2}{9 \times 2} = \frac{2}{18}$$

Then subtract the numerators and place the result over the common denominator. Reduce the fraction to its lowest terms, if possible. In this case, the fraction can't be reduced.

$$\frac{15}{18} - \frac{2}{18} = \frac{15 - 2}{18} = \frac{13}{18}$$

That wasn't so hard!

More subtraction action

To subtract ¼ from ⅔, follow these steps.

☝ Find the lowest common denominator — in this case, 12.

✌ Convert the fractions to those with the lowest common denominator by multiplying each fraction by the number 1 (in the form of a fraction).

👌 Convert ⅔ to 8⁄12:

$$\frac{2}{3} = \frac{2}{3} \times \frac{12 \div 3}{12 \div 3} = \frac{2}{3} \times \frac{4}{4} = \frac{2 \times 4}{3 \times 4} = \frac{8}{12}$$

🖐 Convert ¼ to 3⁄12:

$$\frac{1}{4} = \frac{1}{4} \times \frac{12 \div 4}{12 \div 4} = \frac{1}{4} \times \frac{3}{3} = \frac{1 \times 3}{4 \times 3} = \frac{3}{12}$$

🖐 Subtract the numerators and place the result over the common denominator:

$$\frac{8}{12} - \frac{3}{12} = \frac{8 - 3}{12} = \frac{5}{12}$$

Multiplying fractions

Good news! There's no need to convert to common denominators when multiplying fractions. Simply multiply the numerators and denominators in turn.

For example, to multiply 4⁄7 by 5⁄8, multiply the numerators 4 and 5 and the denominators 7 and 8 to get a new fraction. Here's the calculation.

• Set up the equation:

$$\frac{4}{7} \times \frac{5}{8}$$

• Multiply the numerators and multiply the denominators:

$$\frac{4 \times 5}{7 \times 8} = \frac{20}{56}$$

• Reduce the answer to its lowest terms:

$$\frac{5}{14}$$

Let's see it again

To multiply $\frac{5}{6}$ by $\frac{1}{3}$, multiply the numerators 5 and 1 and the denominators 6 and 3 to get the answer:

$$\frac{5}{6} \times \frac{1}{3} = \frac{5 \times 1}{6 \times 3} = \frac{5}{18}$$

A whole other matter

To multiply a fraction by a whole number, for example $\frac{1}{9}$ by 4, follow these simple steps:

• First, convert the whole number 4 to the fraction $\frac{4}{1}$.

• Then multiply the numerators and denominators. The complete calculation looks like this:

$$\frac{1}{9} \times 4 = \frac{1}{9} \times \frac{4}{1} = \frac{1 \times 4}{9 \times 1} = \frac{4}{9}$$

Dividing fractions

In division (as in multiplication), you don't need to convert the fractions. Division problems are usually written as two fractions separated by a division sign. The first fraction is the number to be divided (the dividend), and the second fraction is the number doing the dividing (the divisor):

This fraction is the dividend.

$$\frac{5}{7} \div \frac{2}{3}$$

This fraction is the divisor.

To divide fractions, multiply the dividend by the divisor's reciprocal, or the inverted divisor.

• To divide $\frac{5}{7}$ by $\frac{2}{3}$ (the divisor), first multiply $\frac{5}{7}$ (the dividend) by $\frac{3}{2}$ (the divisor's reciprocal):

$$\frac{5}{7} \div \frac{2}{3} = \frac{5}{7} \times \frac{3}{2}$$

• Then complete the calculation and reduce the answer (the quotient) to its lowest terms:

$$\frac{5 \times 3}{7 \times 2} = \frac{15}{14} = 1\frac{1}{4}$$

A part divided by a whole

To divide a fraction by a whole number, use the same principle.

• To divide $\frac{3}{5}$ by 2, first convert the whole number 2 to the fraction $\frac{2}{1}$.

$$\frac{3}{5} \div 2 = \frac{3}{5} \div \frac{2}{1}$$

- Then multiply the dividend (³⁄₅) by the reciprocal of the divisor (½). Reduce the answer to its lowest terms:

$$\frac{3}{5} \times \frac{1}{2}$$

$$\frac{3 \times 1}{5 \times 2}$$

$$\frac{3}{10}$$

In this case, the answer can't be further reduced.

Making things less complex

In complex fractions, the numerators and denominators are fractions themselves. Complex fractions can be simplified by following the rules for division of fractions. Think of the line separating the two fractions as a division sign. For example, follow the simple steps below to simplify the complex fraction:

$$\frac{\frac{1}{3}}{\frac{5}{8}}$$

 First, rewrite the complex fraction as a division problem:

$$\frac{\frac{1}{3}}{\frac{5}{8}} = \frac{1}{3} \div \frac{5}{8}$$

 Multiply the dividend (⅓) by the reciprocal of the divisor (⁸⁄₅):

$$\frac{1}{3} \times \frac{8}{5}$$

Finally, complete the calculation:

$$\frac{1 \times 8}{3 \times 5} = \frac{8}{15}$$

Cheat sheet

Key points when using fractions

Adding and subtracting
- Always convert to fractions with common denominators first when adding and subtracting fractions.

Multiplying
- Don't convert fractions to common denominators.
- Multiply numerators and denominators in turn.

Dividing
- Don't convert fractions to common denominators.
- Write as two fractions separated by a division sign.
- Invert the divisor.
- Multiply the dividend by the inverted divisor.

Don't forget!
- Always reduce the final answer to its lowest terms.
- If the fraction is improper, convert to a mixed number.

Quick quiz

1. ⅔ × ⁵⁄₇ is:
  A.   ¹⁴⁄₁₅.
  B.   ¹⁰⁄₂₁.
  C.   ⅞.

Answer: B. To multiply two common fractions, multiply the numerators and then the denominators. The calculation looks like this:

$$\frac{2}{3} \times \frac{5}{7} = \frac{2 \times 5}{3 \times 7} = \frac{10}{21}$$

2. In the fraction ⅘, the denominator is:
  A.   4.
  B.   5.
  C.   ⁵⁄₄.

Answer: B. The denominator is the bottom number of a fraction. The numerator is the top number.

3. When you reduce the fraction ⁸⁄₂₄ to its lowest terms, you get:
  A.   ⅖.
  B.   ¾.
  C.   ⅓.

Answer: C. Both the numerator and the denominator are divisible by 8, leaving the reduced fraction ⅓.

4. Which of the following is an improper fraction?
  A.   ⁹⁄₁₇
  B.   1½
  C.   ⅓

Answer: B. An improper fraction has a numerator that's larger than the denominator.

5. When adding the fractions ⅓ and ½, you get:
  A.   ⅚.
  B.   ⅜.
  C.   ⁵⁄₂₀.

Answer: A. To add ½ and ⅓, first find the common denominator, which is 6. Convert the fractions to ³⁄₆ and ²⁄₆. Then add the numerators and place the result over the common denominator. The calculation looks like this:

$$\frac{1}{2} + \frac{1}{3} = \frac{3}{6} + \frac{2}{6} = \frac{3 + 2}{6} = \frac{5}{6}$$

6.   Which of the following is a prime number?
    A.   4
    B.   5
    C.   6

Answer: B. The number 5 is a prime number because it can be divided only by itself and 1.

Scoring

☆☆☆ If you answered all six items correctly, wow! You're a number 1 math whiz (which is the same as a $\frac{2}{2}$ math whiz and a $\frac{3}{3}$ math whiz).

☆☆ If you answered four or five correctly, fantastic! You're a free-wheeling fraction fiend!

☆ If you answered fewer than four correctly, stick with it! You've shown great derring-do in dealing with dividends and divisors.

Decimals and percentages

Just the facts

In this chapter, you'll learn:

♦ what decimals and percentages are

♦ how to add, subtract, multiply, divide, and round off decimal fractions

♦ how to convert common fractions to decimal fractions and vice versa

♦ how to convert percentages to decimal fractions and common fractions and vice versa

♦ how to solve percentage problems.

A look at decimals and percentages

For most people, decimals and percentages are a part of everyday life. Figuring a tip at a restaurant, balancing a checkbook, and interpreting the results of an election or a survey are just three ways people use decimals and percentages.

As a nurse, you also encounter decimals and percentages every day at work. The metric system, the most common system for measuring medications, is based on decimal numbers. You also use decimals and percentages when administering solutions such as 0.9% sodium chloride solution and drugs such as a 2.5% cream.

In the know

To administer medications accurately and efficiently, you must understand what decimals and percentages are and how to work with them in common calculations. You also need to know how to convert from percentages to decimal fractions and common fractions and then back to percentages. This chapter will sharpen your calculation skills and help you build confidence.

Deciphering decimals

A *decimal fraction* is a proper fraction in which the denominator is a power of 10, signified by a decimal point placed at the left of the numerator. An example of a decimal fraction is 0.2, which is the same as ²⁄10.

In a *decimal number*—for example, 2.25—the decimal point separates the whole number from the decimal fraction.

Look to the left...

Each number or place to the left of the decimal point represents a whole number that's a power of 10, starting with ones and working up to tens, hundreds, thousands, ten thousands, and so on.

...and then to the right

Each place to the right of the decimal point signifies a fraction whose denominator is a power of 10, starting with tenths and working up to hundredths, thousandths, ten thousandths, and so on. When working as a nurse, you'll rarely encounter decimal fractions beyond the thousandths. (See *Know your places.*)

Know your places

Based on its position relative to the decimal point, each decimal place represents a power of 10 or a fraction with a denominator that is a power of 10, as shown below.

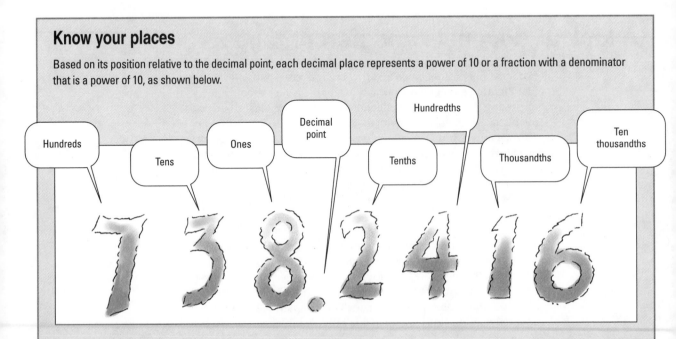

Getting to the point

When discussing money, people use the word *and* to signify the decimal point, for example, saying $5.20 as "5 dollars and 20 cents." However, when discussing decimal numbers in dosage calculations, use the word *point* to signify the decimal point. For example, say the number 5.2 as "5 point 2."

Zeroing in on zeros

Now that you've learned the basic terms used with decimal fractions, you're ready to review the decimal calculations most often performed by nurses. But first, review these two important rules:
• After performing mathematical functions with decimal numbers, you may eliminate zeros to the right of the decimal point that don't appear before other numbers. (See *Zap those zeros*.) In other cases, you may wish to *add* zeros at the end of fractions (for example, as place holders). Deleting or adding zeros at the end of a decimal fraction doesn't change the value of the number.
• When writing answers to mathematical calculations and specifying drug dosages, always put a zero to the left of the decimal point if no other number appears there. This helps prevent errors. (See *Disappearing decimal alert*, page 28.)

Zap those zeros

Are you solving a problem with decimal numbers? In most cases, you can delete all zeros to the right of the decimal point that don't appear before other numbers.

Before you give that drug!

Disappearing decimal alert

Decimal points and zeros may be small items, but they're big deals on medication order sheets and administration records. When you get a drug order, study it closely. If a dose doesn't sound right, maybe a decimal point was left out or incorrectly placed.

For instance, an order that calls for ".5 mg lorazepam I.V." may be mistaken for "5 mg of lorazepam I.V." The correct way to write this order is to use a zero as a placeholder before the decimal point. The order would then become "0.5 mg lorazepam I.V."

Adding and subtracting decimal fractions

Before adding and subtracting decimal fractions, align the decimal points vertically to help you keep track of the decimal positions.

Placeholders, take your place

To maintain column alignment, add zeros as placeholders in decimal fractions.

Here's how to use zeros to align the decimal fractions 2.61, 0.315, and 4.8 before adding:

$$
\begin{array}{r}
2.610 \\
0.315 \\
+\ 4.800 \\
\hline
7.725
\end{array}
$$

Working it out

Here are two more examples of adding and subtracting decimal fractions. First, add 0.017, 4.8, and 1.22:

$$
\begin{array}{r}
0.017 \\
4.800 \\
+\ 1.220 \\
\hline
6.037
\end{array}
$$

Next, subtract 0.05 from 4.726:

$$\begin{array}{r} 4.726 \\ -\ 0.050 \\ \hline 4.676 \end{array}$$

Multiplying decimal fractions

Aligning the decimal points isn't necessary before doing a multiplication problem with decimal fractions. Just leave the decimal points in their original positions.

In the final product, the number of decimal places equals the sum of the decimal places in the numbers being multiplied. In other words, when you arrive at your answer, count the decimal places starting from the right. Then place the decimal point to the left of the last place counted. Here's how you would multiply 2.7 and 0.81:

$$\begin{array}{r} 2.70 \\ \times\ 0.81 \\ \hline 2.1870 \end{array}$$

Multiple multiplication

Here are two more examples of multiplying decimal fractions. First, multiply 1.423 and 8.59:

$$\begin{array}{r} 1.423 \\ \times\ 8.59 \\ \hline 12.22357 \end{array}$$

Next, multiply 42.1 and 0.376:

$$\begin{array}{r} 42.1 \\ \times\ 0.376 \\ \hline 15.8296 \end{array}$$

Dividing decimal fractions

When dividing decimal fractions, align the decimal points but don't add zeros as placeholders. Begin by reviewing the parts of a division problem.

Remember: The number to be divided is the dividend, the number that does the dividing is the divisor, and the answer is the quotient. (See *Divvying up the problem*.)

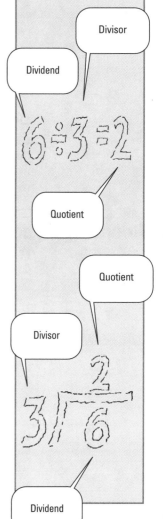

Divvying up the problem

Before you can divide numbers, you need to know what each part of a division problem is called. The division problem below can be written two different ways, but the terms remain the same.

Divisor

Dividend

Quotient

Quotient

Divisor

Dividend

Whole-number divisors

Decimal point placement is easiest when the divisor is a whole number. Just place the decimal point in the quotient directly above the decimal point in the dividend and then work the problem. For example, here's how to divide 4.68 by 2:

$$2\overline{)\,4.68} = 2.34$$

Align decimal points.

Revisiting decimal division

Here are two more examples of decimal point placement when the divisor is a whole number. First, divide 44.02 by 10:

$$10\overline{)\,44.020} = 4.402$$

Next, divide 9.093 by 3:

$$3\overline{)\,9.093} = 3.031$$

Align decimal points.

Decimal-fraction divisors

Of course, not every divisor is a whole number — some are decimal fractions. Dividing one decimal fraction into another requires moving the decimal points in both the divisor and the dividend. (See *Dividing decimal fractions.*)

Rounding off decimal fractions

Most of the instruments and measuring devices a nurse uses measure accurately only to a tenth or, at most, to a hundredth. So you'll need to round off decimal fractions — that is, convert long fractions to those with fewer decimal places. (See *Remember rounding*, page 32.)

Whittling decimals down

To round off a decimal fraction, follow these steps:

☞ Suppose you want to round off the decimal fraction 0.4293. First, decide how many places to the right of the decimal point you want to keep. If you decide to round the number off to hundredths, you'll keep two places to the right of the decimal point and delete the rest (the 9 and the 3).

✌ Now, look at the first number that you've deleted. Is this number 5 or greater than 5? If so, add 1 to the number in the hun-

Cheat sheet

Key points when using decimals

Adding and subtracting
• Align the decimal points vertically.
• Use zeros to maintain column alignment.

Multiplying
• Don't move decimal points.
• The number of decimal places in the product equals the sum of decimal places in the numbers multiplied.

Dividing
• When a whole number is the divisor, place the quotient's decimal point directly above the dividend's decimal point.
• When a decimal fraction is the divisor, move the divisor's decimal point to the right to convert to a whole number, move the dividend's decimal point the same number of places to the right, place the quotient's decimal point directly above the dividend's decimal point.

For math phobics only

Dividing decimal fractions

When dividing one decimal fraction by another, move the divisor's decimal point all the way to the right to convert it to a whole number. Move the dividend's decimal point the same number of places to the right. After completing the division problem, place the quotient's decimal point directly above the new decimal point in the dividend.

The example below shows how to divide 10.45 by 2.6. The quotient is rounded to the nearest hundredth.

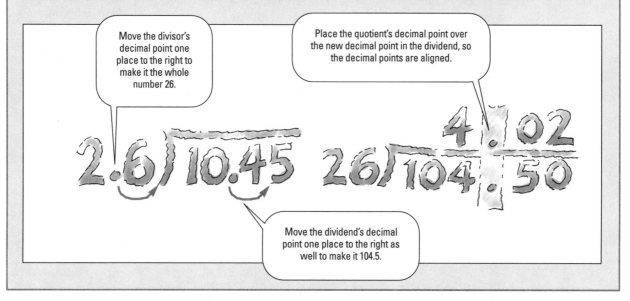

Move the divisor's decimal point one place to the right to make it the whole number 26.

Place the quotient's decimal point over the new decimal point in the dividend, so the decimal points are aligned.

Move the dividend's decimal point one place to the right as well to make it 104.5.

dredths place — that is, to the number 2. Your rounded-off number is now 0.43.

Suppose the number that you delete is less than 5. Then don't add 1 to the number on the left. For example, to round off 1.9085 to the nearest tenth, identify the number in the tenths position (9) and delete all the numbers to the right of it (0, 8, and 5). Because the number directly to the right of 9 — the 0 — is less than 5, the number 9 stays the same. The number 1.9085 rounded off to the nearest tenth is 1.9.

A practice round

Try rounding off 14.723 to the nearest hundredth:
• First, decide what number is in the hundredths place (2) and delete all the numbers to the right of it (only the number 3).
• Because 3 is lower than 5, you don't add 1 to the 2. Thus, the rounded-off number is 14.72.

Now, round off 0.9875 to the nearest thousandth:
• The number in the thousandth place is 7. All numbers to the right of the 7 — the 5 — will be deleted.
• Because the number to be deleted is a 5, the 7 is rounded *up* to 8 (7 + 1). The rounded-off number is therefore 0.988.

Converting fractions

Many measuring devices have metric calibrations, so you'll often need to convert common fractions to decimal fractions. At times, you may also need to convert decimal fractions back into common fractions.

Converting common fractions to decimal fractions

Changing a common, proper fraction into a decimal fraction is simple. Just divide the numerator by the denominator. Add a zero as a placeholder to the left of the decimal point.

Commence converting

For example, here's how to convert ⁴⁄₁₀ to a decimal fraction:

$$\text{⁴⁄₁₀} = 4 \div 10 = 10\overline{)4.0}^{\,0.4}$$

Keep on converting

Here are two more examples. First, convert ²⁄₅ to a decimal fraction:

$$\text{²⁄₅} = 2 \div 5 = 5\overline{)2.0}^{\,0.4}$$

Next, convert ³⁄₈ to a decimal fraction:

$$\text{³⁄₈} = 3 \div 8 = 8\overline{)3.000}^{\,0.375}$$

Converting mixed numbers to decimal fractions

How do you convert a mixed number to a decimal fraction? First, convert it to an improper fraction and then divide the numerator by the denominator, as shown above.

that's easy,
6.45
2.99
4.12

Mixing it up

Here's an example. To convert 4¾ to a decimal fraction, first convert the mixed number 4¾ to the improper fraction, ¹⁹⁄₄. Then divide 19 by 4 to find the decimal fraction:

$$4¾ = ¹⁹⁄₄ = 19 \div 4 = 4\overline{)19.00}^{\,4.75}$$

Let's see that again

Here are two more calculations to try. First, convert 10⅞ to a decimal fraction:

$$10⅞ = ⁸⁷⁄₈ = 87 \div 8 = 8\overline{)87.00}^{\,10.88}$$

Next, convert 1²⁄₉ to a decimal fraction:

$$1²⁄₉ = ¹¹⁄₉ = 11 \div 9 = 9\overline{)11.00}^{\,1.22}$$

Converting decimal fractions to common fractions

To convert a decimal fraction to a common fraction, count the number of decimal places in the decimal fraction. This number reflects the number of zeros in the denominator of the common fraction.

For example, to convert the decimal fraction 0.33 into a common fraction, follow these steps.

☝ Count the number of decimal places in 0.33. There are two decimal places, so the denominator of its common fraction is 100 because 100 has two zeros.

✌ Remove the decimal point from 0.33 and use this number as the numerator. Reduce the fraction, if possible.

The calculation looks like this:

$$0.33 = \frac{33}{100}$$

This fraction can't be reduced further.

You need not have an aversion to conversion. It can be incredibly easy!

Practice, practice, practice

Try two more calculations. First, convert 0.413 to a common fraction. Here, the denominator is 1,000 because the decimal fraction (0.413) has three places after the decimal point.

The calculation looks like this:

$$0.413 = \frac{413}{1,000}$$

This fraction can't be reduced further.

Now convert 0.65 to a common fraction. The denominator is 100 because this decimal fraction has two places after the decimal point.

The calculation looks like this:

$$0.65 = \frac{65}{100} = \frac{13}{20}$$

Note that this fraction has been reduced to its lowest terms.

Converting decimal fractions to mixed numbers

Use the same method as described previously to convert a decimal fraction to a mixed number (or to an improper fraction).

Mixed up but methodical

For example, to convert 5.75 to a fraction, use 100 as the denominator because 5.75 has two decimal places. Then convert the fraction to a mixed number.

The calculation looks like this:

$$5.75 = \frac{575}{100} = 5\frac{75}{100} = 5\frac{3}{4}$$

Note that this mixed number has been reduced to its lowest terms.

That was beautiful! Do it again

Below are two more sample calculations. First, convert 3.25 to a fraction. Use 100 as the denominator because 3.25 has two decimal places. Then convert the fraction to a mixed number.

The calculation looks like this:

$$3.25 = \frac{325}{100} = 3^{25}/_{100} = 3\frac{1}{4}$$

Note that this mixed number has been reduced.

Once more and you got it

Convert 1.9 to a fraction. Use 10 as the denominator because 1.9 has one decimal place. Then convert the fraction to a mixed number.

The calculation looks like this:

$$1.9 = \frac{19}{10} = 1\frac{9}{10}$$

Note that this mixed number can't be further reduced.

Understanding percentages

Percentages are another way to express fractions and numerical relationships. The percent symbol may be used with a whole number such as 21%, a mixed number such as 34½%, a decimal number such as 0.9%, or a fraction such as ⅛%. (See *A point about percents*.)

From discounts to drug doses

You use percentages in everyday life when figuring department store discounts or restaurant tips. You also use them in nursing when calculating solutions and drug doses. Because percentages are such an important part of your work, you must know how to convert easily from percentages to decimal fractions and common fractions and vice versa.

A point about percents

When you see %, the percent sign, think "for every hundred." Why? Because percentage means any quantity stated as parts per hundred. In other words, 75% is actually ⁷⁵/₁₀₀ because the percent sign takes the place of the denominator 100.

Converting percentages to decimals

To change a percentage to a decimal fraction, remove the % sign and multiply the number in the percentage by ¹/₁₀₀, or 0.01. For example, you would convert 84% and 35% to decimal fractions in this way:

$$84 \times 0.01 = 0.84$$

$$35 \times 0.01 = 0.35$$

Watch that decimal point

Make sure that you shift the decimal point in the right direction (to the left, when converting a percentage to a decimal); otherwise you could calculate a drug dose incorrectly. (See *From percentages to decimals [and back again]*, page 36.)

Converting percentages to common fractions

Suppose you want to convert 50% to a common fraction. To convert a percentage to a common fraction, follow these steps:

For math phobics only

From percentages to decimals (and back again)

Although it seems like a harmless dot, a misplaced decimal point can lead to a serious drug error. Study the examples below to see how to perform conversions quickly and accurately.

Jump to the left

To convert from a percentage to a decimal, remove the percent sign and move the decimal point two places to the *left*. Here's how:

$$97\% = 0.97$$

> Remove the percent sign and move the decimal point two places to the left.

Jump to the right

To convert a decimal to a percentage, reverse the process. Move the decimal point two places to the *right*; add a zero as a placeholder, if necessary; and then add a percent sign. If the resulting percentage is a whole number, remove the decimal because it's understood. Here's what the calculation looks like:

$$0.20 = 20\%$$

> Move the decimal point two places to the right and add a percent sign.

- First, remove the percent sign and put the decimal point two places to the left, creating the decimal fraction 0.50:

$$50\% = 0.50$$

- Next, convert 0.50 to a common fraction with a denominator that's a factor of 10. The result is $^{50}/_{100}$ because 0.50 has two decimal places:

$$0.50 = \frac{50}{100}$$

- Finally, reduce the fraction to its lowest terms, which is ½:

$$\frac{50}{100} = \frac{1}{2}$$

so,

$$50\% = \frac{1}{2}$$

Incredible! Do it again!

Here's another example. To convert 32.7% to a common fraction, remove the percent sign and put the decimal point two places to the left, creating the decimal fraction 0.327. Convert 0.327 to a common fraction using 1,000 as the denominator because 0.327 has three decimal places:

$$32.7\% = 0.327 = \frac{327}{1,000}$$

The result is ³²⁷⁄₁,₀₀₀, a fraction that's already reduced to its lowest terms.

Again?

All right, here's one last example: To convert 20.05% to a common fraction, remove the percent sign and put the decimal point two places to the left, creating the decimal fraction 0.2005. Use 10,000 as the denominator because 0.2005 has four decimal places:

$$20.02\% = 0.2005 = \frac{2,005}{10,000} = \frac{401}{2,000}$$

The result is ²,⁰⁰⁵⁄₁₀,₀₀₀, which becomes ⁴⁰¹⁄₂,₀₀₀ when reduced.

Converting common fractions to percentages

Converting a common fraction to a percentage involves two simple steps. Suppose you want to convert ⅖ to a decimal. First, divide the numerator, 2, by the denominator, 5. You can do this by hand or with a calculator. (See *Thank heaven for calculators*.)

Thank heaven for calculators

A calculator can simplify converting a common fraction to a decimal fraction. For example, to convert a mixed number like 2⅘ to a decimal fraction, first convert it to the improper fraction ¹⁴⁄₅. Then follow these steps on the calculator:

 Enter the numerator, 14.

 Press ÷.

 Enter the denominator, 5.

 Press = to obtain the converted number, 2.8.

The calculation looks like this:

$$\frac{2}{5} = 2 \div 5 = 5\overline{)2.0}^{\,0.4}$$

Next, convert the decimal fraction to a percentage by moving the decimal point two places to the right (you'll need to add a 0 as a placeholder) and then adding the percent sign.

Here's what the calculation looks like:

$$0.40 = 40\%$$

More practice to make you perfect

Here's a second example. To convert ⅓ to a percentage, create a decimal fraction by dividing 1 by 3. Round off the quotient to two decimal places:

$$\frac{1}{3} = 1 \div 3 = 0.333 = 0.33$$

Then convert the decimal fraction to a percentage by moving the decimal point two places to the right and adding the percent sign:

$$0.33 = 33\%$$

Once more to be sure

Here's a third example. To convert ⅜ to a percentage, create a decimal fraction by dividing 3 by 8:

$$\frac{3}{8} = 3 \div 8 = 0.375$$

Then convert the decimal fraction to a percentage by moving the decimal point two places to the right and adding the percent sign.

The result is:

$$0.375 = 37.5\%$$

Solving percentage problems

Solving percentage problems involves three types of calculations. They are:

- finding a percentage of a number
- finding what percentage one number is of another
- finding a number when a percentage of it is known.

Cheat sheet

Percentages and conversions

Percentages to decimals
- Multiply the percentage number by ¹⁄₁₀₀ (or 0.01).
- Or, shift the decimal two places to the left.

Decimals to percentages
- Divide the decimal fraction by ¹⁄₁₀₀ (or 0.01).
- Or, shift the decimal two places to the right.

Percentages to common fractions
- Remove the percent sign.
- Move the decimal point two places to the left.
- Convert to a common fraction.

Common fractions to percentages
- Divide the numerator by the denominator.
- Convert to a percentage.

You'll have an easier time solving these calculations if you follow a few simple guidelines. (See *Percentage problems: Watch the wording*, page 41.)

Finding a percentage of a number

The question "What is 40% of 200?" is an example of the first type of calculation. To solve it, change the word *of* to a multiplication sign. This gives you:

$$40\% \times 200 = ?$$

Next, convert 40% to a decimal fraction by removing the percent sign and moving the decimal point two places to the left. This gives you:

$$40\% = 0.40$$

Then multiply the two numbers to get the answer, 80:

$$0.40 \times 200 = 80$$

> 40% of 200 is 80.

Practice time (again)

Now, try solving the problem, "What is 5% of 150?" First, restate it as a multiplication problem:

$$5\% \times 150 = ?$$

Next, convert 5% to the decimal fraction 0.05:

$$5\% = 0.05$$

Then multiply the two numbers to get the answer, 7.5:

$$0.05 \times 150 = 7.5$$

> 5% of 150 is 7.5.

Therefore, 7.5 is 5% of 150.

More practice (and you thought the piano was rough)

Here's one more example: "What is 7% of 300?" First, restate the question as a multiplication problem:

$$7\% \times 300 = ?$$

Convert 7% to the decimal fraction 0.07:

$$7\% = 0.07$$

Then multiply the two numbers to get the answer, 21:

$$0.07 \times 300 = 21$$

> 21 is 7% of 300.

Finding what percentage one number is of another

The question "10 is what percentage of 200?" is an example of this type of calculation. To solve it, restate the question as a division problem, with the number 10 as the dividend and the number 200 as the divisor. Here's how the calculation looks so far:

$$200\overline{)10.00}^{\,0.05}$$

Now, move the decimal point in the quotient two places to the right and add a percent sign:

$$0.05 = 5\%$$

> 10 is 5% of 200.

Again (with a twist)

This type of problem can also be expressed in this way: "What percentage of 28 is 14?" To solve it, restate the question as a division problem by making 28 the divisor and 14 the dividend:

$$28\overline{)14.00}^{\,0.50}$$

Then move the decimal point two places to the right and add a percent sign:

$$0.50 = 50\%$$

> 14 is 50% of 28.

One more time

Here's one last problem: "What percentage of 30 is 6?" First, restate the question as a division problem by making 30 the divisor and 6 the dividend:

$$30\overline{)6.00}^{\,0.20}$$

Move the decimal point two places to the right and add a percent sign:

$$0.20 = 20\%$$

> 6 is 20% of 30.

What to do with the remainder

Sometimes, when determining what percentage one number is of another number, the divisor won't divide exactly into the dividend. In these cases, state the quotient as a mixed number by turning the remainder — the undivided part of the quotient — into a common fraction.

Here's how to do this using the problem, "3 is what percentage of 11?"

Restate the question as a division problem, making 11 the divisor and 3 the dividend. Work out the quotient to two places; then take the remainder 3 and make it the numerator of a fraction with the divisor 11 as the denominator.

Here's what the calculation looks like:

$$
\begin{array}{r}
0.27 \\
11\overline{)3.00} \\
2.2 \\
\hline
80 \\
77 \\
\hline
3
\end{array}
$$

The remainder as a common fraction is ³⁄11.

Move the decimal point in the quotient two places to the right and add a percent sign. (The remaining fraction, ³⁄11, is placed to the left of the percent sign.)

$$0.27 \text{ and } ³⁄11 = 27³⁄11\%$$

Back to practice

Let's try a second problem: "5 is what percent of 22?"

Restate the question as a division problem, leaving the remainder after two places as a common fraction:

$$
\begin{array}{r}
0.22 \\
22\overline{)5.00} \\
4\ 4 \\
\hline
60 \\
44 \\
\hline
16
\end{array}
$$

The remainder as a common fraction is ¹⁶⁄22 (reduce to ⁸⁄11).

Move the decimal point in the quotient two places to the right and add a percent sign:

$$0.22⁸⁄11 = 22⁸⁄11\%$$

Just can't get enough of those mixed number quotients

Here's the last example: "13 is what percentage of 45?" Restate the question as a division problem, leaving the remainder after two places as a common fraction:

$$
\begin{array}{r}
0.28 \\
45\overline{)13.00} \\
9\ 0 \\
\hline
4\ 00 \\
3\ 60 \\
\hline
40
\end{array}
$$

Percentage problems: Watch the wording

When a percentage problem is worded this way: "What is 25% of 80?" mentally change the *of* to a multiplication sign so the problem becomes "What is 25% (or, using a decimal fraction, .25) × 80?" Then continue with the calculation. (The answer is 20.)

If a problem is worded as "25 is what percentage of 80?" treat the *what* as a division sign so the problem becomes ²⁵⁄80. Then continue with the calculation. (The answer is 0.3125, or 31.25%.)

The remainder as a common fraction $^{40}/_{45}$ is (reduced to $^8/_9$).
Move the decimal point in the quotient two places to the right
and add a percent sign:

$$0.28^8/_9\% = 28^8/_9\%$$

Finding a number when you know a percentage of it

The third type of problem, finding a number when you know a
percentage of it, also requires division. For example, consider the
following question: "70% of what number is 7?" Here's how to do
this calculation.

First, convert 70% into a decimal fraction by removing the percent sign and moving the decimal point two places to the left:

$$70\% = 0.70$$

Next, divide 7 by 0.70. Move the decimal point two places to
the right in both the divisor (to make it a whole number) and the
dividend. The quotient is 10:

$$0,70\overline{)7,00}^{\;10.}$$

> 70% of 10
> is 7.

Do you feel perfect yet?

Now try the problem "30% of what number is 90?" To solve it, convert 30% to a decimal fraction by removing the percent sign and
moving the decimal point two places to the left:

$$30\% = 0,30$$

Then divide 90 by 0.30. Move the decimal point two places to
the right in both the divisor (to make it a whole number) and the
dividend. The quotient is 300.

$$0,30\overline{)90,000}^{\;300.0}$$

> 30% of 300
> is 90.

Now you're getting the hang of it

Here's a third example: "70% of what number is 28?" To solve this
problem, convert 70% to a decimal fraction by removing the percent sign and moving the decimal point two places to the left:

$$70\% = 0,70$$

Then divide 28 by 0.70. Move the decimal point two places to the right in both the divisor (to make it a whole number) and the dividend. The quotient is 40:

$$0.70{\overline{\smash{)}28.00\,0}} = 40.0$$

> 70% of 40 is 28.

Quick quiz

1. 16% of 79 is:
   A.   0.20
   B.   4.16
   C.   12.64

Answer: C. To solve this, restate the question as a multiplication problem. Convert 16% to a decimal fraction by removing the percent sign and moving the decimal point two places to the left. The decimal fraction is 0.16. Then multiply 0.16 by 79.

2. In the decimal fraction 1.2058, the number in the tenths place is:
   A.   2
   B.   0
   C.   1

Answer: A. The tenths place is to the immediate right of the decimal point.

3. When 3% is converted to a decimal fraction, it becomes:
   A.   0.03
   B.   0.30
   C.   3.0

Answer: A. Remove the percent sign and move the decimal point two places to the left.

4. Converting the common fraction ⅛ to a percentage yields:
   A.   12.5%
   B.   8%
   C.   1/8%

Answer: A. To obtain 12.5, divide 1 by 8; then convert the answer to a percentage by moving the decimal point two places to the right.

5. The decimal fraction 1.9 divided by 3.2 yields:
    A.   0.59
    B.   1.5
    C.   10.55

Answer: A. To solve this, move the decimal points of both the divisor and the dividend one place to the right before dividing. Place the quotient's decimal point over the new decimal point in the dividend.

6. Multiplying 4.9 by 10.203 yields the product:
    A.   49.9947
    B.   49994.7
    C.   0.499947

Answer: A. When multiplying, the number of decimal places in the final product equals the sum of the decimal places in the numbers being multiplied. Count the decimal places starting from the right and place the decimal point there.

Scoring

☆☆☆ If you answered all six items correctly, that's 100% (or 6/6 or, if you prefer decimal fractions, 1.00).

☆☆ If you answered four or five correctly, excellent! As they say, 4/6 to 5/6 ain't bad.

☆ If you answered fewer than four correctly, here's what to do: Subtract the number you got right from 6 and add the result back to your score. Now you've got 100%. Reward yourself with a new calculator!

3

Ratios, fractions, proportions, and solving for *X*

Just the facts

In this chapter, you'll learn:

♦ the definitions of ratios and proportions

♦ how to set up proportions using ratios and fractions

♦ how to solve for *X* in an equation

♦ how ratios, proportions, and solving for *X* relate to dosage calculations.

A look at numerical relationships

Ratios, fractions, and proportions describe relationships between numbers. Ratios use a colon between the numbers in the relationship, as in 4 : 9. Fractions use a slash between numbers in the relationship, as in ⁴/₉.

Proportions are statements of equality between two ratios. For example, to show that 4 : 9 is equal to 8 : 18, you would write:

$$4:9::8:18$$

or

$$\frac{4}{9} = \frac{8}{18}$$

Three major problem solvers

When calculating dosages, you'll use ratios, fractions, and proportions frequently. You'll also use them to perform many other related tasks, such as calculating I.V. infusion rates, converting weights between systems of measurement and, in specialty settings, performing oxygenation and hemodynamic calculations. But before you can use ratios, fractions, and proportions, you need to know how to develop and express them appropriately.

Ratios and fractions

Ratios and fractions are numerical ways to compare items.

Dare to compare

If 100 syringes come in 1 box, then the number of syringes compared to the number of boxes is 100 to 1. This can be written as the ratio 100 : 1 or as the fraction $^{100}/_1$.

On the other hand, the number of boxes to syringes would be 1 : 100 or the fraction $^{1}/_{100}$, so pay attention to which item is mentioned first.

Here are two more examples.

If a hospital's critical care area requires 1 registered nurse for every 2 patients, then the relationship of registered nurses to patients is 1 to 2. You can express this with the ratio 1 : 2 or with the fraction $^{1}/_2$.

Or, suppose a vial has 8 mg of a drug in 1 ml of solution. By using a ratio, you can express this as 8 mg : 1 ml. By using a fraction, you can describe it as $^{8\,mg}/_{1\,ml}$.

Proportions

Any proportion that's expressed as two ratios also can be expressed as two fractions.

Using ratios in proportions

When using ratios in a proportion, separate them with double colons. Double colons represent equality between the two ratios.

For example, if the ratio of syringes to boxes is 100 : 1, then 200 syringes are provided in 2 boxes. This proportion can be written as:

100 syringes : 1 box :: 200 syringes : 2 boxes

or

100 : 1 :: 200 : 2

Proportion practice

Here's another example. If the critical care area has 1 nurse for every 2 patients, you can express this as the ratio 1 : 2. You can also say that this equals a ratio of 3 nurses for every 6 patients. In a proportion, you can express this relationship with the ratios:

$$1 \text{ nurse} : 2 \text{ patients} :: 3 \text{ nurses} : 6 \text{ patients}$$

or

$$1 : 2 :: 3 : 6$$

Another portion of proportions

Now, suppose you have a vial that contains 8 mg of a drug in 1 ml of a solution. You can state this as the ratio 8 mg : 1 ml, which equals 16 mg : 2 ml. This proportion can be expressed with ratios as follows:

$$8 \text{ mg} : 1 \text{ ml} :: 16 \text{ mg} : 2 \text{ ml}$$

or

$$8 : 1 :: 16 : 2$$

Using fractions in proportions

Any proportion that can be expressed with ratios can also be expressed with fractions. Here's how to do this using the previous examples.

If 100 syringes come in a box, this means that 200 syringes come in 2 boxes. Using fractions, you can write this proportion as:

$$\frac{100 \text{ syringes}}{1 \text{ box}} = \frac{200 \text{ syringes}}{2 \text{ boxes}}$$

or

$$\frac{100}{1} = \frac{200}{2}$$

Fraction action

If the critical care area has 1 nurse for every 2 patients, this means that it has 3 nurses for every 6 patients. Using fractions, you can express this relationship as:

$$\frac{1 \text{ nurse}}{2 \text{ patients}} = \frac{3 \text{ nurses}}{6 \text{ patients}}$$

or

$$\frac{1}{2} = \frac{3}{6}$$

Working out ratios, fractions, and proportions puts you in good shape for dosage calculations.

Vial trial run

If there are 8 mg of a drug in 1 ml, this means there are 16 mg in 2 ml. This proportion can be expressed with fractions as:

$$\frac{8 \text{ mg}}{1 \text{ ml}} = \frac{16 \text{ mg}}{2 \text{ ml}}$$

or

$$\frac{8}{1} = \frac{16}{2}$$

Solving for *X*

We know that a proportion is a set of two equal ratios or fractions. But what if one ratio or fraction is incomplete? In this case, the unknown part of the ratio or fraction is represented by *X*. You can solve for *X* to determine the value of the unknown quantity. (See *An explanation of* X.)

Solving common-fraction equations

The method used to solve common-fraction equations forms the basis for solving other types of simple equations to find the value of *X*. For example, here's how to solve the common-fraction equation:

$$X = \frac{1}{5} \times \frac{3}{9}$$

 Multiply the numerators:

$$1 \times 3 = 3$$

 Multiply the denominators:

$$5 \times 9 = 45$$

 Restate the equation with this new information:

$$X = \frac{1 \times 3}{5 \times 9} = \frac{3}{45}$$

What does it all mean?

An explanation of X

Being able to find the value of X is vital in making dosage calculations. For example, suppose a doctor orders a drug for your patient, but the drug isn't available in the ordered strength. How do you decide on the right amount of drug to administer?

Here's how

Suppose you receive an order to administer 0.1 mg of epinephrine subcutaneously, but the only epinephrine on hand is a 1-ml ampule that contains 1 mg of epinephrine. To calculate the volume for injection, state the problem in a proportion:

$$1 \text{ mg} : 1 \text{ ml} :: 0.1 \text{ mg} : X \text{ ml}$$

Rewrite the problem as an equation by applying the principle that the product of the means (numbers in the middle of the proportion) equals the product of the extremes (numbers at the end of the proportion).

$$1 \text{ ml} \times 0.1 \text{ mg} = 1 \text{ mg} \times X \text{ ml}$$

Solve for X by dividing both sides of the equation by the known value that appears on the same side of the equation as the unknown value X. Then cancel out units that appear in the numerator and denominator. (This isolates X on one side of the equation.)

$$\frac{1 \text{ ml} \times 0.1 \text{ mg}}{1 \text{ mg}} = \frac{1 \text{ mg} \times X \text{ ml}}{1 \text{ mg}}$$

$$X = 0.1 \text{ ml}$$

Reduce the fraction by dividing the numerator and denominator by the lowest common denominator (3), to find that $X = \frac{1}{15}$.

$$X = \frac{3 \div 3}{45 \div 3} = \frac{1}{15}$$

Most dosage calculations require your answer to be in decimal form, so convert $\frac{1}{15}$ to a decimal fraction by dividing the numerator by the denominator. Round the answer off to the nearest hundredth. The final result is $X = 0.07$.

$$X = \frac{1}{15} = 1 \div 15 = 0.07$$

Try this X-ample

Now, solve for X in the equation:

$$X = \frac{2}{3} \times \frac{5}{8}$$

Memory jogger

The term X-factor is often used to describe a person or event that could cause unexpected, or unknown, outcomes. Keep this in mind and you'll remember that X represents the unknown part of a ratio or fraction.

Multiply the numerators:

$$2 \times 5 = 10$$

Multiply the denominators:

$$3 \times 8 = 24$$

Restate the equation with this new information:

$$X = \frac{2 \times 5}{3 \times 8} = \frac{10}{24}$$

Reduce the fraction by dividing the numerator and denominator by the lowest common denominator (2), to find that $X = \frac{5}{12}$.

$$X = \frac{10 \div 2}{24 \div 2} = \frac{5}{12}$$

Convert $\frac{5}{12}$ to a decimal fraction by dividing the numerator by the denominator and then rounding it off. The final result is $X = 0.42$.

$$X = \frac{5}{12} = 5 \div 12 = 0.42$$

Here comes a curveball

This example has a twist — the whole number 3 is involved. (See *Making whole numbers fractions.*)

This is how to solve for *X* in an equation with a whole number:

$$X = \frac{125}{500} \times 3$$

Convert the whole number 3 into the fraction $\frac{3}{1}$. The equation becomes:

$$X = \frac{125}{500} \times \frac{3}{1}$$

Next, reduce $\frac{125}{500}$ by dividing the numerator and denominator by the lowest common denominator (125) to get $\frac{1}{4}$. The equation becomes:

$$X = \frac{125 \div 125}{500 \div 125} \times \frac{3}{1}$$

or

$$X = \frac{1}{4} \times \frac{3}{1}$$

Then proceed as usual. Multiply the numerators:

$$1 \times 3 = 3$$

Multiply the denominators:

$$4 \times 1 = 4$$

Restate the equation with this new information:

$$X = \frac{1 \times 3}{4 \times 1} = \frac{3}{4}$$

The fraction ¾ can't be reduced. Convert it to a decimal fraction by dividing the numerator by the denominator. The final result is $X = 0.75$.

$$X = \frac{3}{4} = 3 \div 4 = 0.75$$

For math phobics only

Making whole numbers fractions

You can change any whole number into a fraction by making the whole number the numerator and placing it over a 1, which is the denominator. The value of the number doesn't change.

Numerator

Whole number

Denominator

Slip a 1 under here.

Solving decimal-fraction equations

To solve for X in equations with decimal fractions, use a method similar to that used above. This is how to solve for X in the equation:

$$X = \frac{0.05}{0.02} \times 3$$

Remove the decimal points from the fraction by moving them two spaces to the right. Then remove the zeros. The equation becomes:

$$X = \frac{5}{2} \times 3$$

Next, convert the whole number 3 to the fraction ³⁄₁. The equation becomes:

$$X = \frac{5}{2} \times \frac{3}{1}$$

Then multiply the numerators:

$$5 \times 3 = 15$$

Multiply the denominators:

$$2 \times 1 = 2$$

Restate the equation with this new information:

$$X = \frac{5 \times 3}{2 \times 1} = \frac{15}{2}$$

Convert the answer to decimal form by dividing 15 by 2. The final result is $X = 7.5$.

$$X = \frac{15}{2} = 15 \div 2 = 7.5$$

X-tra credit

Here's another practice problem:

$$X = \frac{0.33}{0.11} \times 0.6$$

You won't be decimated by decimal-fraction equations!

Remove the decimal points from the fraction by moving them two spaces to the right. Then remove the zeros. The equation becomes:

$$X = \frac{33}{11} \times 0.6$$

Convert the number 0.6 into the fraction $^{0.6}/1$. The equation becomes:

$$X = \frac{33}{11} \times \frac{0.6}{1}$$

Multiply the numerators:

$$33 \times 0.6 = 19.8$$

Multiply the denominators:

$$11 \times 1 = 11$$

Restate the equation with this new information:

$$X = \frac{33 \times 0.6}{11 \times 1} = \frac{19.8}{11}$$

Convert the answer to decimal form by dividing 19.8 by 11. The final result is $X = 1.8$.

$$X = \frac{19.8}{11} = 19.8 \div 11 = 1.8$$

All this practice is beginning to pay off!

X-tra, X-tra credit

Here's the last problem:

$$X = \frac{0.04}{0.05} \times 4$$

Remove the decimal points from the fraction by moving them two places to the right. Then delete the zeros. The equation becomes:

$$X = \frac{4}{5} \times 4$$

Turn 4 into the fraction ⁴⁄₁. The equation becomes:

$$X = \frac{4}{5} \times \frac{4}{1}$$

 Multiply the numerators:

$$4 \times 4 = 16$$

 Multiply the denominators:

$$5 \times 1 = 5$$

 Restate the equation with this new information:

$$X = \frac{4 \times 4}{5 \times 1} = \frac{16}{5}$$

 Convert the answer to decimal form by dividing 16 by 5. The final answer is $X = 3.2$.

$$X = \frac{16}{5} = 16 \div 5 = 3.2$$

Solving proportion problems with ratios

A proportion can be written with ratios, as in:

Extreme

Mean

$$4:1::20:5$$

Extreme

Mean

The outer or end numbers are called the *extremes*, and the inner or middle numbers are called the *means*. In such a proportion, the product of the means equals the product of the extremes. In this case,

The product of the means…

$$1 \times 20 = 4 \times 5$$

…equals the product of the extremes

This principle lets you solve for any of four unknown parts in a proportion.

X marks another spot

Here's an example. Solve for *X* in the proportion:

$$4:8::8:X$$

Follow these steps:

 Rewrite the problem so that the means and the extremes are multiplied:

$$8 \times 8 = 4 \times X$$

 Obtain the products of the means and extremes and put them into an equation:

$$64 = 4X$$

 Solve for *X* by dividing both sides by 4. Cancel the number (4) that appears in both the numerator and denominator. This isolates *X* on one side of the equation.

$$\frac{64}{4} = \frac{\cancel{4}X}{\cancel{4}}$$

Find *X*:

$$64 \div 4 = X$$

or

$$X = 16$$

Replace *X* with 16 and restate the proportion in ratios:

$$4:8::8:16$$

X moves back to the front

Solve for *X* in the proportion:

$$X:12::6:24$$

Follow these steps:

Arrrgh! That darn X keeps moving around!

SNAP

Rewrite the problem so that the means and the extremes are multiplied:

$$12 \times 6 = X \times 24$$

 Obtain the products of the means and extremes and put them into an equation:

$$72 = 24X$$

Finding *X*

Common-fraction equations
• Multiply numerators.
• Multiply denominators.
• Restate the equation.
• Reduce the fraction.

Decimal-fraction equations
• Move the decimal points two spaces to the right.
• Remove the zeros.
• Convert the whole number to a fraction.
• Multiply the numerators.
• Multiply the denominators.
• Restate the equation.
• Convert the answer to decimal form by dividing the numerator by the denominator.

Proportions with ratios
• Extremes—end numbers
• Means—middle numbers
• Product of the means = product of the extremes

 Solve for *X* by dividing both sides by 24. Cancel the number (24) that appears in both the numerator and denominator. This isolates *X* on one side of the equation:

$$\frac{72}{24} = \frac{24X}{24}$$

 Find *X*:

$$72 \div 24 = X$$

or

$$X = 3$$

Replace *X* with 24 and restate the proportion in ratios:

$$3 : 12 :: 6 : 24$$

Another X-treme shift

Try one last problem, using this proportion:

$$10 : 20 :: X : 40$$

Rewrite the problem so that the means and the extremes are multiplied:

$$20 \times X = 10 \times 40$$

Obtain the products of the means and extremes and put them into an equation:

$$20X = 400$$

 Solve for *X* by dividing both sides by 20. Cancel the number (20) that appears in both the numerator and denominator. This isolates *X* on one side of the equation:

$$\frac{20X}{20} = \frac{400}{20}$$

Find *X*:

$$X = \frac{400}{20}$$

or

 $$X = 20$$

Replace *X* with 20 and restate the original proportion in ratios:

$$10:20::20:40$$

Solving proportion problems with fractions

Proportion problems may also be set up with fractions. In a proportion expressed as a fraction, cross products are equal — just as the means and extremes are equal in a proportion with ratios. (See *Cross product principle*.)

What does it all mean?

Cross product principle

In a proportion expressed as fractions, cross products are equal. In other words, the numerator on the equation's left side multiplied by the denominator on the equation's right side equals the denominator on the equation's left side multiplied by the numerator on the equation's right side.

The above statement has a lot of words. The same meaning is communicated more simply in the following illustration.

Applies to ratios as well

Note that the same principle applies to ratios. In a proportion expressed as ratios, the product of the **means** (numbers in the middle) equals the product of the **extremes** (numbers on the **ends**.) Consider the illustration to the right.

Using the cross products of a proportion, you can solve for any of four unknown parts. Once again, the position of the *X* doesn't matter because the cross products of a proportion are always equal. (See *Cross products to the rescue.*)

Keeping things in proportion

After studying the example in *Cross products to the rescue*, practice solving for *X* using this proportion:

$$\frac{3}{4} = \frac{9}{X}$$

Follow these steps:

 Rewrite the problem so the cross products are multiplied:

$$3 \times X = 4 \times 9$$

 Obtain the cross products and put them into an equation:

$$3X = 36$$

For math phobics only

Cross products to the rescue

Fractions can be used to describe the relative proportion of ingredients, for example, the amount of a drug relative to its solution.

Suppose you have a vial containing 10 mg/ml of morphine sulfate. You can write this fraction to describe it:

Amount of drug

$$\frac{10\ mg}{1\ ml}$$

Amount of solution

The plot thickens

Now suppose you want to administer 8 mg of morphine sulfate to your patient. How much of the solution should you use?

1. Write a second fraction using *X* to represent the amount of solution:

$$\frac{8\ mg}{X\ ml}$$

An unknown quantity

2. Set up the equation. Keep the fractions in the same relative proportion of drug to solution.

3. Rewrite the problem so cross products are multiplied:

Cross multiply

$$\frac{10\ mg}{1\ ml} \diagdown \frac{8\ mg}{X\ ml}$$

4. This gives you:

$$10X = 8$$

5. Solve for *X* by dividing both sides by 10, and you're left with:

$$X = \frac{8}{10}$$

6. Convert this to a decimal fraction because you'll be drawing up medication and need to work with a decimal:

$$X = 0.8\ ml$$

The answ

This is how much of the morphine sulfate you should use.

Solve for *X* by dividing both sides by 3. Cancel the number (3) that appears in both the numerator and denominator. This isolates *X* on one side of the equation:

$$\frac{3X}{3} = \frac{36}{3}$$

Find *X*:

$$X = \frac{36}{3}$$

or

$$X = 12$$

Replace the *X* with 12 and restate the proportion in fractions:

$$\frac{3}{4} = \frac{9}{12}$$

Final practice problem (Yippee!)

Solve one more problem:

$$\frac{12}{25} = \frac{X}{50}$$

Rewrite the problem so the cross products are multiplied:

$$12 \times 50 = 25 \times X$$

Obtain the cross products and put them into an equation:

$$600 = 25X$$

Solve for *X* by dividing both sides by 25:

$$\frac{600}{25} = \frac{25X}{25}$$

Find *X*:

$$X = 24$$

Replace *X* with 24 and restate the proportion in fractions:

$$\frac{12}{25} = \frac{24}{50}$$

Real world problems

Next, you'll find three practical examples of proportions in everyday nursing practice.

How do you set up a proportion to solve a real world problem? Just place the known ratio on one side of the double colon and the unknown ratio on the other side. Be sure that the units of measure in each ratio are in the same positions on both sides of the proportion. (See *Write it down.*)

How much hydrogen peroxide?

Set up a proportion to find out how much hydrogen peroxide (H_2O_2) you should add to 1,000 ml of water (H_2O) to make a solution that contains 50 ml of H_2O_2 for every 100 ml of H_2O.

The ratio approach

To solve this problem using ratios, follow these steps:

☝ Decide what part of the ratio is *X*. In this case, it's the amount of H_2O_2 in 1,000 ml of H_2O.

✌ Set up the proportion so that similar parts of each ratio are in the same position:

$$X : 1{,}000 \text{ ml } H_2O :: 50 \text{ ml } H_2O_2 : 100 \text{ ml } H_2O$$

🖐 Multiply the means and the extremes and restate the problem as an equation:

$$1{,}000 \text{ ml } H_2O \times 50 \text{ ml } H_2O_2 = X \text{ ml } H_2O_2 \times 100 \text{ ml } H_2O$$

🖐 Solve for X by dividing both sides of the equation by 100 ml H_2O and canceling units that appear in both the numerator and denominator:

$$\frac{1{,}000 \cancel{\text{ ml } H_2O} \times 50 \text{ ml } H_2O_2}{100 \cancel{\text{ ml } H_2O}} = \frac{X \text{ ml } H_2O_2 \times 100 \cancel{\text{ ml } H_2O}}{100 \cancel{\text{ ml } H_2O}}$$

🖐 Find *X*:

$$\frac{50{,}000 \text{ ml } H_2O_2}{100} = X$$

or

$$X = 500 \text{ ml } H_2O_2$$

The fraction approach

If you set up a proportion with fractions, place similar units of measure for each fraction in the same position. Here's what the previous example looks like in fraction form:

$$\frac{X}{1{,}000 \text{ ml } H_2O} = \frac{50 \text{ ml } H_2O_2}{100 \text{ ml } H_2O}$$

 Rewrite the equation by cross-multiplying the fractions:

$$X \times 100 \text{ ml } H_2O = 1{,}000 \text{ ml } H_2O \times 50 \text{ ml } H_2O_2$$

 Solve for X by dividing both sides of the equation by 100 ml H_2O and canceling units that appear in both the numerator and denominator:

$$\frac{X \times \cancel{100 \text{ ml } H_2O}}{\cancel{100 \text{ ml } H_2O}} = \frac{1{,}000 \cancel{\text{ ml } H_2O} \times 50 \text{ ml } H_2O_2}{100 \cancel{\text{ ml } H_2O}}$$

 Find X:

$$X = \frac{50{,}000 \text{ ml } H_2O_2}{100}$$

$$X = 500 \text{ ml } H_2O_2$$

How many clinical instructors?

Set up another proportion problem with both ratios and fractions. If a school of nursing requires 1 clinical instructor for every 8 students, how many instructors are needed for a class of 24 students?

Resolving it with ratios

Use ratios first. Follow these steps:

 Decide what part of the proportion is X. In this case, it's the number of instructors for 24 students.

 Set up the proportion so that the units of measure (instructors and students) in each ratio are in the same position:

1 instructor : 8 students :: X : 24 students

 Multiply the means and the extremes and set up the equation:

8 students $\times X$ = 1 instructor $\times$ 24 students

See all that fractions and ratios can do?

Solve for *X* by dividing both sides of the equation by 8 students and canceling units that appear in both the numerator and denominator:

$$\frac{8\ \cancel{students} \times X}{8\ \cancel{students}} = \frac{1\ \text{instructor} \times 24\ \cancel{students}}{8\ \cancel{students}}$$

Find *X*:

$$X = 3\ \text{instructors}$$

Figuring it out with fractions

If you prefer to solve the previous problem using fractions, follow these steps:

Set up the proportion so that the units of measure are in the same position in each fraction. Here's what the problem looks like in fraction form:

$$\frac{1\ \text{instructor}}{8\ \text{students}} = \frac{X}{24\ \text{students}}$$

Rewrite the equation by cross-multiplying the fractions:

1 instructor × 24 students = *X* instructors × 8 students

Solve for *X* by dividing both sides of the equation by 8 students and canceling units that appear in both the numerator and denominator:

$$\frac{1\ \text{instructor} \times 24\ \cancel{students}}{8\ \cancel{students}} = \frac{X \times 8\ \cancel{students}}{8\ \cancel{students}}$$

or

$$24 \div 8 = X\ \text{instructors}$$

Find *X*:

$$X = 3\ \text{instructors}$$

How many bags of I.V. fluid?

Here's one more problem. One case of I.V. fluid holds 20 bags. If your home care agency receives 6 cases, how many bags of I.V. fluid does it have?

The ratio rally

Solve this problem using ratios first. Follow these steps:

 Decide what part of the ratio is X. In this case, it's the number of bags of I.V. fluid in 6 cases.

Set up the proportion so that the units of measure in each ratio are in the same position:

$$1 \text{ case} : 20 \text{ bags} :: 6 \text{ cases} : X$$

Multiply the means and the extremes and set up the equation:

$$20 \text{ bags} \times 6 \text{ cases} = X \text{ bags} \times 1 \text{ case}$$

Solve for X by dividing both sides of the equation by 1 case and canceling units that appear in both the numerator and denominator:

$$\frac{20 \text{ bags} \times 6 \text{ cases}}{1 \text{ case}} = \frac{X \times \text{1 case}}{\text{1 case}}$$

Find X.

$$120 \text{ bags} = X$$

The fraction finale

Now, use fractions to solve the problem. Here's what the equation looks like in fraction form:

$$\frac{1 \text{ case}}{20 \text{ bags}} = \frac{6 \text{ cases}}{X}$$

Rewrite the equation by cross-multiplying the fractions. Then solve for X by dividing each side of the equation by 1 case and canceling units that appear in both the numerator and denominator:

$$\frac{\text{1 case} \times X}{\text{1 case}} = \frac{6 \text{ cases} \times 20 \text{ bags}}{1 \text{ case}}$$

$$X = 120 \text{ bags}$$

Quick quiz

1. An example of a proportion is:
   A.   4 : 5 :: 8 : 12
   B.   6 : 1 :: 18 : 3
   C.   7 : 1 :: 14 : 7

Answer: B. In a proportion, the ratios are equal.

2. In fraction form, the proportion 1 : 5 :: 2 : 10 is:
   A. $\frac{1}{5} = \frac{2}{10}$
   B. $\frac{5}{1} = \frac{2}{10}$
   C. $\frac{2}{5} = \frac{1}{10}$

Answer: A. Make the ratios on both sides into fractions by substituting slashes for colons.

3. If there are 50 mg of a drug in 5 ml of solution, the amount of drug in 15 ml of solution is:
   A.   10 mg
   B.   150 mg
   C.   75 mg

Answer: B. Substitute X for the amount of drug in 15 ml of solution and then set up a proportion with ratios or fractions.

4. The amount of salt you should add to 32 oz of water to make a solution with ½ (0.5) tsp of salt for every 8 oz of water is:
   A.   2 tsp
   B.   4 tsp
   C.   1 tsp

Answer: A. Substitute X for the amount of salt in 32 oz of water and then set up a proportion with ratios or fractions.

Scoring

☆☆☆ If you answered all four items correctly, wow! You're a whiz at relationships (numerical relationships, that is).

☆☆ If you answered two or three correctly, all right! You have everything in proportion.

☆ If you answered fewer than two correctly, a quick review will get your numbers back on track!

Dimensional analysis

Just the facts

In this chapter, you'll learn:

♦ what dimensional analysis is

♦ how to set up an equation using dimensional analysis

♦ how to identify conversion factors

♦ how to solve dosage calculations using dimensional analysis.

A look at dimensional analysis

Dimensional analysis, also known as *factor analysis* or *factor labeling*, is an alternative way of solving mathematical problems. It's a basic and easy approach to calculating drug dosages because it eliminates the need to memorize formulas. Only one equation is required to determine each answer.

Factors are the main actors

When using dimensional analysis, a series of ratios, called *factors*, are arranged in a fractional equation. Each factor, written as a fraction, consists of two quantities of measurement that are related to each other in a given problem. Dimensional analysis uses the same terms as fractions, specifically the terms *numerator* and *denominator*.

Setting the stage

Let's say you want to change 48″ to feet. The problem is written as follows:

$$48'' = X \text{ feet}$$

Some problems contain all of the information needed to identify the factors, set up the equation, and find the solution. Other problems, such as this one, require a conversion factor.

Conversion factors

Conversion factors are equivalents between two units of measurement. For example, 1 day equals 24 hours. In this case, day and hour are units of measurement and, when stated as 1 day = 24 hours, they're equivalent. This conversion factor can be used to solve problems involving the measure of time. There are many commonly used conversion factors. (See *Common conversion factors.*)

Putting it into practice

In the previous problem of how many feet are in 48″, use the conversion factor 12″ equals 1′.

Because the quantities and unit of measurement are equivalent, they can serve as the numerator or denominator. The conversion can be written as:

$$\frac{12}{1}$$

or

$$\frac{1}{12}$$

Setting up the equation

Solving a problem using dimensional analysis is like climbing a staircase — it requires steps. Six simple steps need to be followed to solve any problem. (See *Following the steps.*)

Stepping up to the problem

Let's take it one step at a time:

☝ Given quantity — This is the beginning point of the problem. Identify the given quantity in the problem. In this case,

$$48″$$

✌ Wanted quantity — This is the answer to the problem. Identify the wanted quantity in the problem as an unknown unit. In this problem it's :

$$X \text{ feet}$$

🖖 Conversion factors — Again, these are the equivalents that are necessary to convert between systems. The conversion factor for this problem is :

$$12″ = 1′$$

Advice from the experts

Common conversion factors

Keep this chart handy for quick reference to breeze through problems that call for these common conversions.

1 kg = 2.2 lb
16 oz = 1 lb
8 oz = 1 cup
12″ = 1′
3 = 1 yd

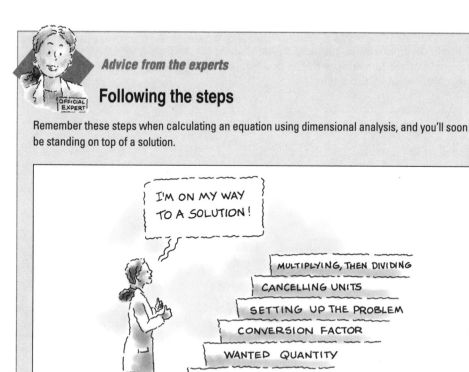

Advice from the experts

Following the steps

Remember these steps when calculating an equation using dimensional analysis, and you'll soon be standing on top of a solution.

Set up the problem using necessary equivalents as conversion factors. You want to cancel the inches and get the answer in feet. To do this, you must multiply 48″ by a fraction that has inches in the denominator and feet in the numerator. The problem should be set up as follows:

$$\frac{48 \text{ inches}}{1} \times \frac{1 \text{ foot}}{12 \text{ inches}}$$

Unwanted units — Just as with any type of mathematical problem, you'll cancel units that appear in both the numerator and denominator to isolate the unit you're seeking. In this case, you'll cancel inches, thereby isolating feet, which is the desired measurement. The step will look like this:

$$\frac{48 \text{ inches}}{1} \times \frac{1 \text{ foot}}{12 \text{ inches}}$$

Multiply the numerators, multiply the denominators, and divide the product of the numerators by the product of the denominators to reach the wanted quantity.

$$\frac{4}{1} \times \frac{1 \text{ foot}}{1} = \frac{4 \times 1 \text{ foot}}{1 \times 1} = \frac{4}{1} = 4 \text{ feet}$$

There are 4′ in 48″.

Let's step to it again

Now try to solve another problem using dimensional analysis. A package weighs 38 oz. How many pounds does it weigh?
- Identify the given:

$$38 \text{ oz}$$

- Identify the wanted:

$$X \text{ pounds}$$

- Identify the conversion factor:

$$1 \text{ lb} = 16 \text{ oz}$$

- Set up the equation:

$$\frac{38 \text{ oz}}{1} \times \frac{1 \text{ lb}}{16 \text{ oz}}$$

- Cancel units that appear in both the numerator and denominator:

$$\frac{38 \cancel{\text{ oz}}}{1} \times \frac{1 \text{ lb}}{16 \cancel{\text{ oz}}}$$

Dimensional analysis works!

- Multiply the numerators and denominators and divide the products:

$$\frac{38 \times 1 \text{ lb}}{1 \times 16} = \frac{38 \text{ lb}}{16} = 2.4 \text{ lb}$$

There are 2.4 lb in 38 oz.

Let's cool down...with one more rep!

Getting a good workout? Try one more to keep in peak shape. If you drank 64 oz of juice, how many cups of juice did you drink?
- Identify the given:

$$64 \text{ oz}$$

- Identify the wanted:

$$X \text{ cups}$$

- Identify the conversion factor:

$$8 \text{ oz} = 1 \text{ cup}$$

- Set up the equation:

$$\frac{64 \text{ oz}}{1} \times \frac{1 \text{ cup}}{8 \text{ oz}}$$

- Cancel units that appear in both the numerator and denominator:

$$\frac{64 \text{ oz}}{1} \times \frac{1 \text{ cup}}{8 \text{ oz}}$$

- Multiply the numerators and denominators and divide the products:

$$\frac{64 \times 1 \text{ cup}}{1 \times 8} = \frac{64 \text{ cups}}{8} = 8 \text{ cups}$$

There are 8 cups in 64 oz.

Take a breath and let's review

Now that you've made it through the steps again, let's pause to study some key ideas. Dimensional analysis is a method of problem solving that can be used whenever two quantities are directly proportional to each other. One of the quantities can be converted to another unit of measurement by using common equivalents or conversion factors. The problem is treated as an equation using fractions.

Now on your feet and do it again!

Apply the concepts you just reviewed above. Tom is taking a 9-mile hike. If he normally walks at a pace of 2.5 miles per hour, how long will it take Tom to do the 9-mile hike?
- Identify the given:

$$9 \text{ miles}$$

- Identify the wanted:

$$X \text{ hours}$$

- Identify the conversion factor:

$$2.5 \text{ miles} = 1 \text{ hour}$$

- Set up the equation:

$$\frac{9 \text{ miles}}{1} \times \frac{1 \text{ hour}}{2.5 \text{ miles}}$$

Cheat sheet

Dimensional analysis

- Use whenever two quantities are directly proportional to each other.
- Use common equivalents or conversion factors to convert to the same unit of measurement.
- Express the problem as an equation with fractions.

• Cancel units that appear in both the numerator and denominator:

$$\frac{9 \ \text{miles}}{1} \times \frac{1 \ \text{hour}}{2.5 \ \text{miles}}$$

• Multiply the numerators and denominators and divide the products:

$$\frac{9 \times 1 \ \text{hour}}{1 \times 2.5} = \frac{9 \ \text{hours}}{2.5} = 3.6 \ \text{hours}$$

It will take Tom 3.6 hours to complete his walk.

Real world problems

A patient is ordered to have 70 mg of enoxaparin (Lovenox). It's available in vials that contain 30 mg per 0.3 ml. How much should be prepared?

• Begin by identifying the given quantity:

$$70 \ \text{mg}$$

• Then isolate what you're looking for:

$$X \ \text{ml}$$

• Know your conversion factor:

$$30 \ \text{mg} = 0.3 \ \text{ml}$$

• Set up the equation:

$$\frac{70 \ \text{mg}}{1} \times \frac{0.3 \ \text{ml}}{30 \ \text{mg}}$$

• Identify and cancel units that appear in both the numerator and denominator:

$$\frac{70 \ \text{mg}}{1} \times \frac{0.3 \ \text{ml}}{30 \ \text{mg}}$$

• Finally, multiply the numerators and denominators and divide the products:

$$\frac{70 \times 0.3 \ \text{ml}}{1 \times 30} = \frac{21 \ \text{ml}}{30} = 0.7 \ \text{ml}$$

The patient would receive 0.7 ml of Lovenox.

Solve for Synthroid

A patient is to receive 50 mcg of levothyroxine (Synthroid). The drug is available as 200 mcg per 5 ml. How many milliliters should the nurse prepare?

Practice really pays off.

- The given quantity:

$$50 \text{ mcg}$$

- The wanted quantity:

$$X \text{ ml}$$

- The conversion factor:

$$200 \text{ mcg} = 5 \text{ ml}$$

- Set up the equation:

$$\frac{50 \text{ mcg}}{1} \times \frac{5 \text{ ml}}{200 \text{ mcg}}$$

- Cancel units that appear in both the numerator and denominator:

$$\frac{50 \ \cancel{\text{mcg}}}{1} \times \frac{5 \text{ml}}{200 \ \cancel{\text{mcg}}}$$

- Then multiply the numerators and denominators and divide the products:

$$\frac{50 \times 5 \text{ ml}}{1 \times 200} = \frac{250 \text{ ml}}{200} = 1.3 \text{ ml}$$

The nurse should prepare 1.3 ml of Synthroid.

How much heparin?

The doctor prescribes 10,000 U of heparin added to 500 ml of D_5W at 1,200 U/hour. How many drops per minute should you administer if the I.V. tubing delivers 10 gtt/ml?

- The given quantities (in this case there are three):

$$\text{1st quantity: } \frac{10 \text{ gtt}}{1 \text{m ml}}$$

$$\text{2nd quantity: } \frac{500 \text{ ml}}{10,000 \text{ U}}$$

$$\text{3rd quantity: } \frac{1,200 \text{ U}}{1 \text{ hour}}$$

- The conversion factor:

$$\frac{1 \text{ hour}}{60 \text{ minutes}}$$

- Set up the equation:

$$\text{gtt/minute} = \frac{10 \text{ gtt}}{1 \text{ ml}} \times \frac{500 \text{ ml}}{10,000 \text{ U}} \times \frac{1,200 \text{ U}}{1 \text{ hour}} \times \frac{1 \text{ hour}}{60 \text{ minutes}}$$

- Cancel the units that appear in both the numerator and denominator:

$$\text{gtt/minute} = \frac{10 \text{ gtt}}{1 \text{ m\!l}} \times \frac{500 \text{ m\!l}}{10,000 \text{ U\!}} \times \frac{1,200 \text{ U\!}}{1 \text{ hour}} \times \frac{1 \text{ hour}}{60 \text{ minutes}}$$

- Then multiply the numerators and denominators and divide the products:

$$\frac{10 \times 500 \times 1,200 \text{ gtt}}{10,000 \times 60 \text{ minutes}} = \frac{6,000,000 \text{ gtt}}{600,000 \text{ minutes}} = 10 \text{ gtt/minute}$$

You should administer the heparin at a rate of 10 gtt/minute.

Lasso the Lasix

Let's try one more problem. Your patient is to receive 20 mg of furosemide (Lasix) oral solution. The bottle is labeled 40 mg per 5 ml. How many milliliters will the patient receive?

- The given quantity:

20 mg

- The wanted quantity:

X ml

- The conversion factor:

40 mg = 5 ml

- Set up the equation:

$$\frac{20 \text{ mg}}{1} \times \frac{5 \text{ ml}}{40 \text{ mg}}$$

- Cancel units that appear in both the numerator and denominator:

$$\frac{20 \cancel{\text{ mg}}}{1} \times \frac{5 \text{ ml}}{40 \cancel{\text{ mg}}}$$

- Multiply the numerators and denominators and divide the products:

$$\frac{20 \times 5 \text{ ml}}{1 \times 40} = \frac{100 \text{ ml}}{40} = 2.5 \text{ ml}$$

The patient would receive 2.5 ml of Lasix oral solution.

Quick quiz

1. When using dimensional analysis, factors are written as:
    A. fractions.
    B. whole numbers.
    C. percentages.

Answer: A. Factors are always written as common fractions. When a problem includes a quantity and its unit of measurement is unrelated to any other factor in the problem, that quantity serves as the numerator of the fraction, and 1 (which is implied) becomes the denominator.

2. The conversion factors in a dimensional analysis equation are:
    A. identified as the given quantity and the wanted quantity.
    B. equivalents necessary to convert between two systems.
    C. always placed as numerators.

Answer: B. Conversion factors involve the use of equivalent measurements that allow for conversion between different systems.

3. Dimensional analysis involves math calculations that can be solved:
  A.   in three simple steps.
  B.   in a single equation.
  C.   using formulas that must be memorized.

Answer: B. When learning dimensional analysis, a step-by-step approach is used, but the problem can be simplified in one single equation.

4. Your patient is 60″ tall. How much is this in feet?
  A.   6′
  B.   6′ 3″
  C.   5′

Answer: C. Use the conversion factor 12″ equals 1′. Then set up the equation and follow the steps:

$$\frac{60 \ \cancel{\text{inches}}}{1} \times \frac{1 \text{ foot}}{12 \ \cancel{\text{inches}}}$$

$$\frac{60 \times 1 \text{ foot}}{1 \times 12} = \frac{60 \text{ feet}}{12} = 5 \text{ feet}$$

5. How many pounds are there in 48 oz?
  A.   4 lb
  B.   3 lb
  C.   5 lb

Answer: B. Use the conversion factor 16 oz equals 1 lb. Then set up the equation and follow the steps:

$$\frac{48 \ \cancel{\text{oz}}}{1} \times \frac{1 \text{ lb}}{16 \ \cancel{\text{oz}}}$$

$$\frac{48 \times 1 \text{ lb}}{1 \times 16} = \frac{48 \text{ lb}}{16} = 3 \text{ lb}$$

Scoring

☆☆☆   If you answered all five items correctly, congratulations! You've added an impressive dimension to your intellect!

☆☆   If you answered three or four items correctly, label yourself a factor to be reckoned with! Don't convert to lazy ways; keep up the good work.

☆   If you answered fewer than three items correctly, please retrace your steps to discover where you went wrong. You'll soon be the equivalent of an expert!

Part II

Measurement systems

5 Metric system   77

6 Alternative measurement systems   91

Metric system

Just the facts

In this chapter, you'll learn:

♦ metric units of measure

♦ how to convert measurements from one metric unit to another

♦ how to solve basic arithmetic problems in metric units

♦ how to calculate drug dosages using the metric system.

A look at the metric system

Today, most nations of the world rely on the metric system of measurement. It's also the most widely used system for measuring amounts of drugs.

The metric system is a decimal system. That means it's based on the number 10 and multiples of 10. The metric system offers three advantages over other systems:
• It eliminates common fractions.
• It simplifies the calculation of large and small units.
• It simplifies the calculation of drug doses. (See *Tips for going metric*, page 78.)

Beginning with the basics

The three basic units of measurement in the metric system (along with the abbreviation for each) are the meter (m), liter (L), and gram (g):
• The meter is the basic unit of length.
• The liter is the basic unit of volume — it's equivalent to $\frac{1}{10}$ of a cubic meter.
• The gram is the basic unit of weight — it represents the weight of 1 cubic centimeter (cm^3 or cc) of water at 4° C (39.2° F.)

What's in a name?

All other units of measure are based on these three major units. When you see the root word *meter*, *liter*, or *gram* within a measurement, you can easily tell if you're measuring length, volume, or weight.

For example, centi*meter* (cm) and milli*meter* (mm) are units of length, centi*liter* (cl) and milli*liter* (ml) are units of volume, and kilo*gram* (kg) and milli*gram* (mg) are units of weight.

Measure for measure

Three devices — the metric ruler, the metric graduate, and metric weights — are used to measure meters, liters, and grams. (See *Measuring meters, liters, and grams.*)

Building on the basics

Multiples and subdivisions of meters, liters, and grams are indicated by using a prefix before the basic unit. Each prefix that's used in the metric system represents a multiple or subdivision of 10.

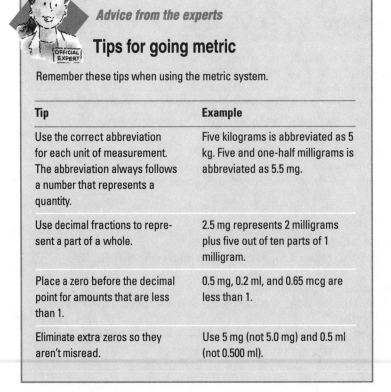

Advice from the experts

Tips for going metric

Remember these tips when using the metric system.

Tip	Example
Use the correct abbreviation for each unit of measurement. The abbreviation always follows a number that represents a quantity.	Five kilograms is abbreviated as 5 kg. Five and one-half milligrams is abbreviated as 5.5 mg.
Use decimal fractions to represent a part of a whole.	2.5 mg represents 2 milligrams plus five out of ten parts of 1 milligram.
Place a zero before the decimal point for amounts that are less than 1.	0.5 mg, 0.2 ml, and 0.65 mcg are less than 1.
Eliminate extra zeros so they aren't misread.	Use 5 mg (not 5.0 mg) and 0.5 ml (not 0.500 ml).

Meters, liters, and grams. I can build on that foundation!

Consider the gram. The most common multiple of a gram is the *kilo*gram, which is 1,000 times greater than the gram. The most common subdivision of a gram is the *milli*gram, which represents ¹⁄₁,₀₀₀ of a gram, or 0.001 g.

Keeping it brief

Any metric measurement can be represented by a number and an abbreviation that represents the unit of measure. The abbreviation stands for the basic unit of measure — gram (g), meter (m), liter (L) — and the prefix, such as kilo (k), centi (c), and milli (m). For example, *kg* stands for kilogram, *cm* for centimeter, and *ml* for milliliter. (See *What a little prefix can do*, page 80.)

A cubic curiosity

The metric system also includes one unusual unit of volume — the cubic centimeter (cc). Because a cubic centimeter occupies the same space as 1 ml of liquid, the two units of volume are considered equal and may be used interchangeably. However, cubic cen-

Measuring meters, liters, and grams

What tools do you need to measure meters, liters, and grams? The appropriate measuring devices, of course. A metric ruler, which resembles a yardstick, is used to measure length. A metric graduate can be used to measure the volume of a fluid in liters. (An enclosed chamber, such as a cylinder with a tight-fitting lid, is needed to measure a volume of gas.) A set of metric weights can be used with a metric balance to measure weight in grams.

Metric graduate

Metric weights

Portion of metric ruler, with inches (upper scale) and centimeters (lower scale)

What a little prefix can do

In the metric system, the addition of a prefix to one of the basic units of measure indicates a multiple or subdivision of that unit. Here's a list of prefixes, abbreviations, and multiples and subdivisions of each unit.

Prefix	Abbreviation	Multiples and subdivisions
kilo	k	1,000
hecto	h	100
deka	dk	10
deci	d	0.1 (1/10)
centi	c	0.01 (1/100)
milli	m	0.001 (1/1,000)
micro	mc	0.000001 (1/1,000,000)
nano	n	0.000000001 (1/1,000,000,000)

timeters usually refer to gas volumes, and milliliters usually describe liquid volumes.

Failing to meet standards

The International Bureau of Weights and Measures adopted the International System of Units in 1960 to promote the standard use of metric abbreviations and prevent errors in drug transcriptions. Unfortunately, some health care providers still use the old abbreviations.

So stay alert for nonstandard abbreviations, especially l instead of L to represent liters, and gm or GM instead of g to represent grams. As a precaution, some nurses and doctors use L in all liter-related abbreviations, such as mL and dL. However, this isn't required.

Metric conversions

Because the metric system is decimal based, converting from one metric unit to another is easy. To convert a smaller unit to a larger unit, move the decimal point to the left. To convert a larger unit to a smaller unit, move the decimal point to the right.

Because all metric units are multiples or subdivisions of the major units, you can also convert a smaller unit to a larger unit by dividing by the appropriate multiple or multiplying by the appropriate subdivision. To convert a larger unit to a smaller unit, multiply by the appropriate multiple or divide by the appropriate subdivision.

Turning to the tables

Luckily, there are tables you can turn to for help in quickly converting measurements. (See *Insta-metric conversion table* and *Amazing metric decimal place finder*, page 82.)

Converting meters to kilometers

Suppose you want to convert 15 meters (m) to kilometers (km). There are two ways to get this done.

Dancing decimal

Using the *Amazing metric decimal place finder*, page 82, you can follow these steps:

Cheat sheet

Metric conversions

Smaller to larger unit
• Move the decimal point to the left.
• Or divide by the appropriate multiple.
• Or multiply by the appropriate subdivision.

Larger to smaller unit
• Move the decimal point to the right.
• Or multiply by the appropriate multiple.
• Or divide by the appropriate subdivision.

Insta-metric conversion table

Want a quick and easy way to jump back and forth between different metric measures? Just use the fantastic "insta-metric" table below. Make a copy of it to post in a conspicuous spot on your unit. And always remember, a milliliter is to a liter as a microgram is to a milligram.

Liquids	Solids
1 ml = 1 cm³ (or cc)	1,000 mcg = 1 mg
1,000 ml = 1 L	1,000 mg = 1 g
100 cl = 1 L	100 cg = 1 g
10 dl = 1 L	10 dg = 1 g
10 L = 1 dkl	10 g = 1 dkg
100 L = 1 hl	100 g = 1 hg
1,000 L = 1 kl	1,000 g = 1 kg

Amazing metric decimal place finder

When performing metric conversions, use the following scale as a guide to decimal placement. Each bar represents one decimal place.

Thousands, Hundreds, Tens, UNITS (GRAMS, LITERS, METERS), Tenths, Hundredths, Thousandths, Ten thousandths, Hundred thousandths, Millionths, Ten millionths, Hundred millionths, Billionths

Kilo, Hecto, Deka, UNITS (GRAMS, LITERS, METERS), Deci, Centi, Milli, Micro, Nano

✌ Count the number of places to the right or left of *meters* to reach *kilo*. You'll see that *kilo* is *three* places to the left, indicating that a kilometer is 1,000 times larger than a meter (note the three zeros in 1,000).

✌ Move the decimal point in 15.0 three places to the *left*, creating the number 0.015. So, 15 m = 0.015 km. *Remember to place a zero in front of the decimal point to draw attention to the decimal point's presence.*

On another road to conversion

Another way to complete this conversion is to use the chart in *What a little prefix can do*, page 80. First, find *kilo*. You'll see that it indicates a multiple of 1,000. When using this chart to go from smaller units to larger units (as you're doing with meters to kilometers), you divide by the multiple.

Here's why: 1 meter multiplied by 1,000 equals 1 km. Think of driving in Europe or Canada, where road distance is measured in kilometers; if you drive 1 m of a 1-km road, you're $\frac{1}{1,000}$ of the way there. Therefore, 1 m equals $\frac{1}{1,000}$ km.

To convert 15 m to kilometers, divide by 1,000. You might want to set up a simple equation:

$$X = \frac{15\,\text{m}}{1,000}$$

$$X = 0.015\,\text{km}$$

So, 15 m = 0.015 km, or 15 thousandths of a kilometer.

Converting grams to milligrams

Now let's say that you want to convert 5 g to milligrams. Again, you can use one of two methods.

Decimal dances again

Using the *Amazing metric decimal place finder,* follow these steps:

Count the number of places to the right or left of *grams* it takes to reach *milli.* You'll see that *milli* is three places to the right, indicating that a milligram is 1,000 times smaller than a gram (note the three zeros in 1,000).

Move the decimal point in 5.0 three places to the right, creating the number 5,000. So 5 g = 5,000 mg.

The multiplying subdivision

Or, as before, the chart in *What a little prefix can do,* page 80, can help you complete your conversion. This time, find *milli.* You'll see that its subdivision is 0.001, or $\frac{1}{1,000}$. When using this table to go from a larger unit to a smaller unit (such as grams to milligrams), divide by the subdivision. Here's why: 1 milligram is $\frac{1}{1,000}$ of a gram. Therefore, 1 g equals 1,000 mg. If you divide 1 g by the subdivision ($\frac{1}{1,000}$), you get 1,000 mg (dividing by $\frac{1}{1,000}$ is the same as multiplying by 1,000). So to convert 5 g to milligrams, divide 5 g by $\frac{1}{1,000}$ (or multiply it by 1,000).

$$X = \frac{5\,\text{g}}{\frac{1}{1,000}}$$

$$X = 5\,\text{g} \times 1,000$$

$$X = 5,000\,\text{mg}$$

As you can see, 5 g = 5,000 mg.

Converting centiliters to liters

How do you convert 350 cl to liters? Here's how using both charts.

Dancing decimal never rests

Using the *Insta-metric conversion table*, page 81, follow these steps:

✍ Count the number of places to the right or left of *centi* it takes to reach *liters*. You'll see that *liters* is two places to the left, indicating that a liter is 100 times larger than a centiliter.

✌ To show this, move the decimal point in 350.0 two places to the left, creating the number 3.5. So, 350 cl = 3.5 L.

Another vision of subdivision

Now refer to the chart in *What a little prefix can do*, page 80. First, find *centi*. You'll see that its subdivision is 0.01 or $1/100$. When using this chart to go from a smaller unit to a larger one (centiliters to liters), you multiply by the subdivision.

Here's why: 1 liter equals 100 cl. Therefore, 1 centiliter is $1/100$ L (or 1 liter divided by 100). To convert 350 cl to liters, multiply 350 cl by $1/100$ (which is the same as dividing by 100) to get 3.5 L.

That Amazing metric decimal place finder really is amazing!

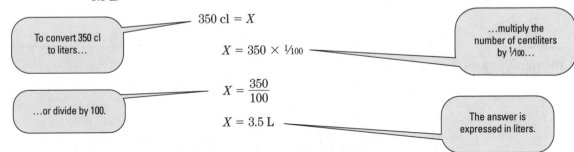

To convert 350 cl to liters...

$$350 \text{ cl} = X$$

$$X = 350 \times 1/100$$

...multiply the number of centiliters by $1/100$...

...or divide by 100.

$$X = \frac{350}{100}$$

$$X = 3.5 \text{ L}$$

The answer is expressed in liters.

Solving for X

Another way to convert between metric units is by solving for X. The following examples show how to solve for X in three clinical situations. If you don't like fractions, see *Overcoming fear of fractions*.

How much does that baby weigh?

An infant weighs 6.5 kg. How much does he weigh in grams? To solve the problem, follow these steps:

For math phobics only

Overcoming fear of fractions

If you don't like working with fractions, here's an alternative to solving for X in problems. In the previous example of determining an infant's weight in grams, the equation that was expressed in fractions can also be set up as a ratio and proportion:

$$1,000 \text{ g} : 1 \text{ kg} :: X : 6.5 \text{ kg}$$

• Multiply the means and extremes:

$$X \times 1 \text{ kg} = 1,000 \text{ g} \times 6.5 \text{ kg}$$

• Divide both sides of the equation by 1 kg to isolate X.
• Cancel units that appear in both the numerator and denominator.

$$X = 6,500 \text{ g}$$

The infant weighs 6,500 g.

First, refer to the *Insta-metric conversion table*, page 81. You'll see that 1,000 g equals 1 kg.

Now set up the following equation, substituting X for the unknown weight in grams:

$$\frac{1,000 \text{ g}}{1 \text{ kg}} = \frac{X}{6.5 \text{ kg}}$$

Cross-multiply the fractions:

$$\frac{1,000 \text{ g}}{1 \text{ kg}} \diagdown\!\!\!\!\!\diagup \frac{X}{6.5 \text{ kg}}$$

$$X \times 1 \text{ kg} = 6.5 \text{ kg} \times 1,000 \text{ g}$$

Divide both sides of the equation by 1 kg to isolate X. Cancel units that appear in both the numerator and denominator:

$$\frac{X \times \cancel{1 \text{ kg}}}{\cancel{1 \text{ kg}}} = \frac{6.5 \cancel{\text{ kg}} \times 1,000 \text{ g}}{1 \cancel{\text{ kg}}}$$

$$X = 6,500 \text{ g}$$

The infant weighs 6,500 g.

> Oh, I remember. *X* stands for the unknown quantity in the equation.

How much I.V. fluid?

If a patient received 0.375 L of lactated Ringer's solution, how many milliliters did he receive?
- Refer to the *Insta-metric conversion table*, page 81. You'll see that 1 L is equal to 1,000 ml.
- Now set up the following equation, substituting X for the unknown amount of I.V. solution in milliliters:

$$\frac{1 \text{ L}}{1,000 \text{ ml}} = \frac{0.375 \text{ L}}{X}$$

- Cross-multiply the fractions:

$$\frac{1 \text{ L}}{1,000 \text{ ml}} \diagdown \frac{0.375 \text{ L}}{X}$$

$$X \times 1 \text{ L} = 0.375 \text{ L} \times 1,000 \text{ ml}$$

- Divide both sides of the equation by 1 L to isolate X. Cancel units that appear in both the numerator and denominator:

$$\frac{X \times \cancel{1 \text{ L}}}{\cancel{1 \text{ L}}} = \frac{0.375 \cancel{\text{ L}} \times 1,000 \text{ ml}}{1 \cancel{\text{ L}}}$$

$$X = 375 \text{ ml}$$

The patient received 375 ml of I.V. fluid.

How much medication?

A nurse administered 2 g of ceftriaxone sodium (Rocephin). How many milligrams of this medication did the patient receive?
- Refer to the *Insta-metric conversion table*, page 81. You'll see that 1 g is equal to 1,000 mg.
- Now set up the following equation, substituting X for the unknown amount of medication in milligrams:

$$\frac{1 \text{ g}}{1,000 \text{ mg}} = \frac{2 \text{ g}}{X}$$

- Cross-multiply the fractions:

$$\frac{1 \text{ g}}{1,000 \text{ mg}} \diagdown \frac{2 \text{ g}}{X}$$

$$X \times 1 \text{ g} = 2 \text{ g} \times 1,000 \text{ mg}$$

- Divide each side of the equation by 1 g, to isolate X. Cancel units that appear in both the numerator and denominator:

$$\frac{X \times \cancel{1g}}{\cancel{1g}} = \frac{2\,g \times 1{,}000\,mg}{1\,g}$$

$$X = 2{,}000\,mg$$

The patient received 2,000 mg of Rocephin.

Metric mathematics

To add, subtract, multiply, or divide different metric units, first convert all quantities to the same unit. Unless the problem calls for an answer in a specific unit, use the common unit that's easiest for you to work with and then perform the arithmetic.

For example, suppose you want to add 2 kg, 202 mg, and 222 g, expressing the total in grams. Here's how to do this:

 First, convert all the measurements to grams. (Refer to the *Insta-metric conversion table*, page 81.)

1 kg equals 1,000 g. Therefore, you can multiply 2 kg by 1,000 to get 2,000 g.

1,000 mg equals 1 g and 1 mg equals $\frac{1}{1{,}000}$ g. Therefore, you can divide 202 mg by 1,000 to get 0.202 g.

Now do the addition:

$$2{,}000 + 0.202 + 222 = 2{,}222.202\,g$$

Real world problems

the Real World

A patient with a 1 L bag of I.V. fluid received 500 ml of fluid over the first shift, 225 ml over the second shift, and 150 ml over the third shift. How many milliliters of fluid remain in the I.V. bag?
• First, determine how much fluid the patient received. To do this, add:

$$500 + 225 + 150 = 875\,ml$$

• Because you're trying to determine the number of milliliters remaining, you only need to convert 1 L to milliliters. Refer to the *Insta-metric conversion table*, page 81 where you'll see that 1 L = 1,000 ml.
• Finally, compute the amount of fluid remaining in the I.V. bag by subtracting 875 ml from 1,000 ml. The answer is 125 ml.

A tantalizing tablet tabulation!

A patient is to receive 5 g of erythromycin (Erythrocin) before intestinal surgery. If erythromycin is available in 500-mg tablets, how many tablets should be administered?
- First, convert all the measures to the same units. Because you're trying to determine the number of 500-mg tablets to administer, convert 5 g to milligrams. Refer to the *Insta-metric conversion table*, page 81, where you'll see that 1 g is equal to 1,000 mg.
- To find how many milligrams are in 5 g, set up this proportion using fractions:

$$\frac{1,000 \text{ mg}}{1 \text{ g}} = \frac{X}{5 \text{ g}}$$

- Then cross-multiply the fractions and divide each side of the resulting equation by 1 g to solve for X:

$$\frac{1,000}{1 \text{ g}} \diagdown \frac{X \text{ mg}}{5 \text{ g}}$$

$$X \times 1 \text{ g} = 1,000 \text{ mg} \times 5 \text{ g}$$

$$\frac{X \times 1\text{g}}{1\text{g}} = \frac{1,000 \text{ mg} \times 5 \text{ g}}{1 \text{ g}}$$

$$X = 5,000 \text{ mg}$$

- You find that X is 5,000 mg.
- To determine the number of 500-mg tablets that need to be administered to provide 5,000 mg, set up another proportion using fractions:

$$\frac{500 \text{ mg}}{1 \text{ tablet}} = \frac{5,000 \text{ mg}}{X}$$

- Cross-multiply the fractions and divide each side of the resulting equation by 500 mg to solve for X:

$$\frac{500 \text{ mg}}{1 \text{ tablet}} \diagdown \frac{5,000 \text{ mg}}{X}$$

$$500 \text{ mg} \times X = 5,000 \text{ mg} \times 1 \text{ tablet}$$

$$\frac{X \times 500\text{ mg}}{500\text{ mg}} = \frac{1 \text{ tablet} \times 5,000 \text{ mg}}{500 \text{ mg}}$$

$$X = 10 \text{ tablets}$$

- You find that X is 10 tablets.
You should administer 10 tablets of erythromycin. (See *Did I get it right?*)

Did I get it right?

There may be times when you work out a dosage calculation and your answer doesn't strike you as being correct. Try verifying your answer by inserting it for X in the equation and doing the calculations. Both sides of the equation should be equal. As an example, let's use the previous problem about erythromycin tablets:

In this problem $X = 10$ tablets, so let's substitute that in the equation for X:

10 tablets = 10 tablets

As you can see, both sides of the equation are equal. Congratulations! You got it right!

Quick quiz

1. Gram, meter, and liter respectively measure:
    A.   length, volume, and weight.
    B.   weight, length, and volume.
    C.   volume, weight, and length.

Answer: B. Gram, meter, and liter — the three basic units of the metric system—measure weight, length, and volume, respectively.

2. According to the International System of Units, the correct abbreviation for gram is:
    A.   gm
    B.   g
    C.   Gm

Answer: B. The standard abbreviation for gram is g.

3. To convert milligrams to grams, move the decimal point:
    A.   three places to the left.
    B.   three places to the right.
    C.   two places to the left.

Answer: A. Locate *milli* and *grams* on the *Amazing metric decimal place finder*, page 82, count the number of places *grams* is to the left of *milli*, and then move the decimal point accordingly.

4. The number of milligrams in 3,120 mcg is:
    A.   3,120,000 mg
    B.   0.312 mg
    C.   3.12 mg

Answer: C. Locate *milli* and *micro* on the *Amazing metric decimal place finder*, page 82, count the number of places *milli* is to the left of *micro*, and then move the decimal point three places to the left.

5. The total volume in milliliters of 312 ml, 3.12 L, and 312 L is:
    A.   327.12 ml
    B.   315,432 ml
    C.   31,543.2 L

Answer: B. Convert all the measures to milliliters and then add all three numbers.

6. The measure that's equivalent to a milliliter is:

    A.   cubic centimeter.

    B.   kiloliter.

    C.   hectoliter.

Answer   A. A milliliter of liquid occupies a cubic centimeter of space.

7. The weight in grams of a baby who weighs 5.2 kg is:

    A.   5.2 g

    B.   5.02 g

    C.   5,200 g

Answer: C. Knowing that 1 kg is equal to 1,000 g, set up an equation with X grams as the unknown quantity and multiply 5.2 kg by 1,000 g/kg.

8. The number of milliliters left in a 4-L bag of normal saline solution after you remove 50 ml, 250 ml, 2.5 L, and 750 ml is:

    A.   3,550 ml

    B.   450 ml

    C.   50 ml

Answer: B. Convert all the measurements to milliliters, add the last four numbers to find out how many milliliters were removed from the bag, and then subtract this number from the amount of fluid in the bag.

9. The smallest metric measurement is the:

    A.   micro.

    B.   deci.

    C.   nano.

Answer: C. The nano, the smallest metric measurement, measures billionths.

Scoring

☆☆☆   If you answered all nine items correctly, give yourself 9 points! If each point were equal to a gram, you'd have 9 grams, or 90 decigrams, or 900 centigrams, or 9,000 milligrams, or 9,000,000 micrograms.

☆☆   If you answered six to eight items correctly, dig those decimals! You're a metric master!

☆   If you answered fewer than six items correctly, leapin' milliliters! Review the chapter again and you'll soon be doing a hecto of a good job!

6

Alternative measurement systems

Just the facts

In this chapter, you'll learn:

♦ what the apothecaries' system is and how it works

♦ what the household system is and how it works

♦ what the avoirdupois system is and how it works

♦ what the unit system is and how it works

♦ what the milliequivalent system is and how it works

♦ how to perform common conversions.

A look at alternative systems

Although the metric system is used most often in clinical settings, you'll work with other systems from time to time. These include the apothecaries', household, avoirdupois, unit, and milliequivalent systems.

When the alternative is the answer...

When would you use these other systems? For example, you might:
- receive a drug order written using the apothecaries' system
- teach a patient to use a measuring device calibrated in the household system
- use the avoirdupois system to calculate a dose that's based on a patient's weight.

You can prepare yourself for these occasions by familiarizing yourself with alternative measurement systems.

Apothecaries' system

Doctors and pharmacists used the apothecaries' system before the metric system was introduced. Since then, use of the older system has declined. But even though this system is rarely seen anymore, you should still be familiar with it.

Basic minims and grains

Unlike the metric system, which is used to measure length, volume, and weight, the apothecaries' system is used to measure only liquid volume and solid weight. The basic unit for measuring liquid volume is the minim, and the basic unit for measuring solid weight is the grain.

Think water and wheat

One way to remember these units is to visualize the minim as about the size of a drop of water, which weighs about the same as a grain of wheat. The following mathematical statement sums up this relationship:

$$1 \text{ drop} = 1 \text{ minim} = 1 \text{ grain}$$

Other units of measure in the apothecaries' system build on these two basic units. Many of these units are also common household measurement. (See *Ye olde apothecaries' system.*)

The dram-a of conversions

Measurements of liquids and solids that are expressed in the apothecaries' system can easily be converted from one unit of measure to another. Here are a few examples:
- How many fluidrams are in 60 minims? From the table shown in *Ye olde apothecaries' system,* you can see that 60 minims equal 1 fluidram.
- How many quarts are in 1 gallon? One gallon equals 4 quarts of fluid.
- How many drams are in 30 grains? Because 60 grains equal 1 dram, 30 grains equal ½ dram.

Roman numerals

Some doctors and pharmacists express apothecaries' system dosages in Arabic numerals followed by units of measure. However, the apothecaries' system traditionally uses Roman numerals. (See *The road to Roman numerals,* page 94.)

Cheat sheet

Apothecaries' system

- Measures liquid volume and solid weight
- Minim—basic unit of liquid volume
- Grain—basic unit of solid weight.
- 1 drop = 1 minim = 1 grain

I prefer to use ye olde calculator!

Ye olde apothecaries' system

The apothecaries' system uses the following units to measure liquid volume and solid weight.

Liquid volume

60 minims = 1 fluidram
8 fluidrams = 1 fluid ounce
16 fluid ounces = 1 pint (pt)
2 pt = 1 quart (qt)
4 qt = 1 gallon (gal)

Solid weight

60 grains (gr) = 1 dram
8 drams = 1 ounce (oz)
12 oz = 1 pound (lb)

When in Rome...

When used in pharmacologic applications, Roman numerals ss (½) through x (10) usually are written in lower case. When Roman numerals are used, the unit of measure goes before the numeral. For example, 5 grains is written grains v. Fractions of less than ½ are written as common fractions using Arabic numerals. Other quantities are expressed by combining letters according to two general rules.

• When a smaller numeral precedes a larger numeral, subtract the smaller numeral from the larger numeral. For example:

$$IX = 10 - 1 = 9$$

• When a smaller numeral follows a larger numeral, add the numerals. For example:

$$XI = 10 + 1 = 11$$

...do as the Romans do!

The road to Roman numerals

Here's a handy review of Roman numerals.

½ = ss	11 = XI	40 = XL
1 = I	12 = XII	50 = L
2 = II	13 = XIII	60 = LX
3 = III	14 = XIV	70 = LXX
4 = IV	15 = XV	100 = C
5 = V	16 = XVI	500 = D
6 = VI	17 = XVII	1,000 = M
7 = VII	18 = XVIII	
8 = VIII	19 = XIX	
9 = IX	20 = XX	
10 = X	30 = XXX	

Breaking up is easy to do

To convert an Arabic numeral to a Roman numeral, first break the Arabic numeral into its component parts; then translate each part into Roman numerals. For example:

$$36 = 30 + 6 = XXX + VI = XXXVI$$

Roman numeral conversions

Now that you understand how Roman numerals work, convert the numbers below.

- Write 53 using Roman numerals:

$$53 = 50 + 3 = L + III = LIII$$

- Write CXXVI using Arabic numerals:

$$CXXVI = C + X + X + VI = 100 + 10 + 10 + 6 = 126$$

- Write 1,558 using Roman numerals:

$$1,558 = 1,000 + 500 + 50 + 8 = M + D + L + VIII = MDLVIII$$

Household system

The household system of measurement uses droppers, teaspoons, tablespoons, and cups to measure liquid medication doses. However, because these measuring devices aren't all alike, the household system is useful only for approximate measurements. For exact measurements, use the metric system. (See *Making sure the cup doesn't runneth over.*)

To measure prescribed drug doses at home, teach the patient the household system. (See *A spoonful of sugar*, page 96.)

Household system conversions

The examples that follow show how to convert measurements using the household system.

> **Teaching points**

Making sure the cup doesn't runneth over

Will your patient be taking medication at home? If so, teach him to use the devices below to help ensure accurate measurements.

Medication cup
A medication cup is calibrated in household, metric, and apothecaries' systems. Tell the patient to set the cup on a counter or flat surface and to check the fluid measurement at eye level.

Dropper
A dropper is calibrated in household or metric systems or in terms of medication strength or concentration. Advise the patient to hold the dropper at eye level to check the fluid measurement.

Hollow-handle spoon
A hollow-handle spoon is calibrated in teaspoons and tablespoons. Teach the patient to check the dose after filling by holding the spoon upright at eye level. Instruct him to administer the medication by tilting the spoon until the medicine fills the bowl of the spoon and then placing the spoon in his mouth.

Cough syrup conundrum

The doctor has ordered 120 drops (gtt) of an expectorant cough syrup every 6 hours for your patient. The drug label gives instructions in teaspoons. How many teaspoons should you administer?
• There are 60 gtt of liquid in 1 teaspoon (tsp). To find out how many teaspoons are in 120 gtt, set up the following equation, using X as the unknown quantity:

$$\frac{60 \text{ gtt}}{1 \text{ tsp}} = \frac{120 \text{ gtt}}{X}$$

• Cross-multiply the fractions:

$$X \times 60 \text{ gtt} = 1 \text{ tsp} \times 120 \text{ gtt}$$

• Solve for X by dividing both sides of the equation by 60 gtt and canceling units that appear in both the numerator and denominator:

$$\frac{X \times \cancel{60 \text{ gtt}}}{\cancel{60 \text{ gtt}}} = \frac{1 \text{ tsp} \times 120 \cancel{\text{ gtt}}}{60 \cancel{\text{ gtt}}}$$

$$X = \frac{1 \text{ tsp} \times 120}{60}$$

$$X = 2 \text{ tsp}$$

The patient should receive 2 tsp of cough syrup.

Broth brain teaser

Your patient is on a clear liquid diet. For lunch he drank 6 tablespoons (tbs) of chicken broth. How many ounces did he consume?
• There are 2 tbs of liquid in 1 ounce (oz). To find out how many ounces are in 6 tbs, set up the following equation, using X as the unknown quantity:

$$\frac{2 \text{ tbs}}{1 \text{ oz}} = \frac{6 \text{ tbs}}{X}$$

• Cross-multiply the fractions:

$$X \times 2 \text{ tbs} = 1 \text{ oz} \times 6 \text{ tbs}$$

• Find X by dividing each side of the equation by 2 tbs and canceling units that appear in both the numerator and denominator:

$$\frac{X \times 2 \cancel{\text{ tbs}}}{2 \cancel{\text{ tbs}}} = \frac{1 \text{ oz} \times 6 \cancel{\text{ tbs}}}{2 \cancel{\text{ tbs}}}$$

$$X = 3 \text{ oz}$$

The patient consumed 3 oz of chicken broth.

Teaching points

A spoonful of sugar

Mary Poppins was no pharmacist, but she knew how to make the medicine go down. She recommended a spoonful of sugar. The question is, how much is in a spoonful?

Here's a rundown of the most commonly used household units of measure and their equivalent liquid volumes. *Note:* Don't use the abbreviations "t" for teaspoon and "T" for tablespoon because it's easy to make errors when writing them quickly.

60 drops (gtt) =
   1 teaspoon (tsp)
3 tsp =
   1 tablespoon (tbs)
2 tbs =
   1 ounce (oz)
8 oz =
   1 cup
16 oz (2 cups) =
   1 pint (pt)
2 pt =
   1 quart (qt)
4 qt =
   1 gallon (gal)

Milk of magnesia mystery

Your patient is to receive 4 tbs of milk of magnesia. This is equal to how many teaspoons?

• There are 3 tsp of liquid in 1 tbs. To find out how many teaspoons are in 4 tbs, set up the following equation using X as the unknown quantity:

$$\frac{3\ \text{tsp}}{1\ \text{tbs}} = \frac{X}{4\ \text{tbs}}$$

• Solve for X by cross-multiplying the fractions, dividing each side of the equation by 1 tbs, and canceling units that appear in both the numerator and denominator:

$$\frac{X \times \cancel{1\ \text{tbs}}}{\cancel{1\ \text{tbs}}} = \frac{3\ \text{tsp} \times 4\ \cancel{\text{tbs}}}{1\ \cancel{\text{tbs}}}$$

$$X = 12\ \text{tsp}$$

The patient gets 12 tsp of milk of magnesia.

Avoirdupois system

This difficult-to-pronounce system of measurement (av-wah-doo-PWAH) is used for ordering and purchasing some pharmaceutical products and for weighing patients.

In this system, the solid measures or units of weight include grains, ounces, and pounds. One ounce equals 480 grains (gr), and 1 lb equals 16 oz or 7,680 gr. Note that the apothecaries' pound equals 12 oz, but the avoirdupois pound equals 16 oz.

Avoirdupois system conversions

The following examples show how to perform conversions in the avoirdupois system:

• How many pounds equal 32 oz? One pound equals 16 oz; therefore, 2 lb equal 32 oz.

• How many ounces equal 7,680 gr? One ounce equals 480 gr; therefore, 16 oz equal 7,680 gr.

• How many gr are in 2 lb? You know that 7,680 gr are in 1 lb; therefore, 15,360 gr are in 2 lb. (See *Measure for measure*, page 98.)

Measure for measure

Here are some approximate liquid and solid equivalents among the household, apothecaries', avoirdupois, and metric systems. Use your facility's protocol for converting measurements from one system to another.

Liquids

Household	Apothecaries'	Metric
1 drop (gtt)	1 minim (m)	0.06 milliliter (ml)
15 to 16 gtt	15 to 16 m	1 ml
1 teaspoon (tsp)	1 fluidram	4 or 5 ml
1 tablespoon (tbs)	½ fluid ounce (oz)	15 or 16 ml
2 tbs	1 fluid oz	30 or 32 ml
1 cup	8 fluid oz	240 or 250 ml
1 pint (pt)	16 fluid oz	473, 480, or 500 ml
1 quart (qt)	32 fluid oz	946, 960, or 1,000 ml (1 liter)
1 gallon (gal)	128 fluid oz	3,785, 3,840, or 4,000 ml

Solids

Avoirdupois	Apothecaries'	Metric
1 grain (gr)	1 gr	0.06 or 0.065 gram (g)
1 gr	1 gr	60 milligrams
15.4 gr	15 gr	1 g
1 oz	480 grains	28.35 g
1 pound (lb)	1.33 lb	454 g
2.2 lb	2.7 lb	1 kilogram (kg)

Unit system

Some drugs are measured in units (U), such as United States Pharmacopoeia (USP) units or International Units (IU). The most common drug that's measured in units is insulin, which comes in such measurements as U-100 strength.

With insulin, the U refers to the number of units per milliliter. For example, 1 ml of U-100 insulin contains 100 units. The U-100 strength, which is based on metric measurements, makes measurement in a standard syringe easy.

Some other drugs are also measured in units, for example, the anticoagulant heparin, the topical antibiotic bacitracin, and penicillins G and V. The hormone calcitonin and the fat-soluble vitamins A, D, and E are measured in IU. Some forms of vitamin A and D are measured in USP units.

All out of proportion

To calculate the dose to be administered when the medication is available in units, use the following proportion:

$$\frac{\text{amount of drug in ml or other measure}}{\text{dose required in U}} = \frac{\text{1 ml or other measure}}{\text{drug available in U}}$$

Cheat sheet

Unit conversions

- Insulin is the most common drug measured in units.
- Divide the units required by the amount of the drug available in units.

Unit system conversions

The examples below show how to perform conversions in the unit system.

Drip...drip...drip...

A standard heparin drip of 25,000 U in 500 ml of half-normal saline solution is ordered for your patient. The heparin vial that's available has 5,000 U/ml. How many milliliters of heparin should you add to the I.V. fluid? This is how to solve this problem:
- Set up a proportion using X as the unknown quantity:

$$\frac{X}{25,000 \text{ U}} = \frac{1 \text{ ml}}{5,000 \text{ U}}$$

- Cross-multiply the fractions:

$$X \times 5,000 \text{ U} = 1 \text{ ml} \times 25,000 \text{ U}$$

- Find X by dividing both sides of the equation by 5,000 U and canceling units that appear in both the numerator and denominator:

$$\frac{X \times \cancel{5,000 \text{ U}}}{\cancel{5,000 \text{ U}}} = \frac{1 \text{ ml} \times 25,000 \cancel{U}}{5,000 \cancel{U}}$$

$$X = 5 \text{ ml}$$

You should add 5 ml of heparin to the I.V. fluid.

Penicillin problem

Your patient needs 500,000 U of penicillin by intramuscular injection. The vial of penicillin that's available contains 1,000,000 U/ml.

How much of the drug should you draw up? This is how to solve this problem.

- Set up a proportion using X as the unknown quantity:

$$\frac{X}{500,000\ U} = \frac{1\ ml}{1,000,000\ U}$$

- Cross-multiply the fractions:

$$X \times 1,000,000\ U = 1\ ml \times 500,000\ U$$

- Find X by dividing each side of the equation by 1,000,000 U and canceling units that appear in both the numerator and denominator:

$$\frac{X \times \cancel{1,000,000\ U}}{\cancel{1,000,000\ U}} = \frac{1\ ml \times 500,000\ \cancel{U}}{1,000,000\ \cancel{U}}$$

$$X = 0.5\ ml$$

You need to inject 0.5 ml of penicillin.

Milliliter mystery

The doctor orders a bolus of 3,000 U of heparin for your patient. The heparin vial that's available contains 1,000 U/ml. How many milliliters should you administer?

- Set up a proportion using X as the unknown quantity of heparin:

$$\frac{X}{3,000\ U} = \frac{1\ ml}{1,000\ U}$$

- Cross-multiply the fractions:

$$X \times 1,000\ U = 1\ ml \times 2,000\ U$$

- Find X by dividing both sides of the equation by 1,000 U and canceling units that appear in both the numerator and denominator:

$$\frac{X \times \cancel{1,000\ U}}{\cancel{1,000\ U}} = \frac{1\ ml \times 2,000\ \cancel{U}}{1,000\ \cancel{U}}$$

$$X = 3\ ml$$

You should administer a 3-ml bolus of heparin.

Milliequivalent system

Electrolytes are measured in milliequivalents (mEq). Drug manufacturers dispense information about the number of metric units required to provide the prescribed number of milliequivalents. For example, the manufacturer's instructions may indicate that 1 ml equals 4 mEq.

A doctor usually orders the electrolyte potassium chloride in milliequivalents. Potassium preparations are available for use in I.V. fluids, as oral suspensions or elixirs, and in solid tablet or powder form. Potassium is also available in the combination drug potassium phosphate. The phosphate in this drug is measured in millimoles.

Cheat sheet

Milliequivalent conversions

- Measures electrolytes
- Divide the amount of milliliters required by the amount of the drug available in milliequivalents.

An propitious proportion

To calculate the dose to be administered when the medication is available in milliequivalents, use the following proportion:

$$\frac{\text{amount of drug in ml or other measure}}{\text{dose required in mEq}} = \frac{\text{1 ml or other measure}}{\text{drug available in mEq}}$$

Milliequivalent system conversions

The problems below show how to do conversions using the milliequivalent system.

Finding the solution for the solution

The doctor has ordered an I.V. infusion of 40 mEq of potassium chloride in 100 ml of normal saline solution for your patient. The potassium vial that's available contains 10 mEq/ml. How many milliliters of potassium chloride should you infuse? This is how to solve this problem.

- Set up a proportion using X as the unknown quantity:

$$\frac{X}{40 \text{ mEq}} = \frac{1 \text{ ml}}{10 \text{ mEq}}$$

- Cross-multiply the fractions:

$$X \times 10 \text{ mEq} = 1 \text{ ml} \times 40 \text{ mEq}$$

- Find X by dividing each side of the equation by 10 mEq and canceling units that appear in both the numerator and denominator:

$$\frac{X \times 10 \text{ mEq}}{10 \text{ mEq}} = \frac{1 \text{ ml} \times 40 \text{ mEq}}{10 \text{ mEq}}$$

$$X = 4 \text{ ml}$$

You need to dilute 4 ml of potassium chloride in the normal saline solution.

Calculate that sodium bicarbonate!

Your patient needs 25 mEq of sodium bicarbonate. The vial from the pharmacy contains 50 mEq in every 50 ml. How many milliliters of the solution should you administer? This is how to solve this problem.

- Set up a proportion using X as the unknown quantity:

$$\frac{X}{25 \text{ mEq}} = \frac{50 \text{ ml}}{50 \text{ mEq}}$$

- Cross-multiply the fractions:

$$X \times 50 \text{ mEq} = 50 \text{ ml} \times 25 \text{ mEq}$$

- Find X by dividing both sides of the equation by 50 mEq and canceling units that appear in both the numerator and denominator:

$$\frac{X \times 50 \text{ mEq}}{50 \text{ mEq}} = \frac{50 \text{ ml} \times 25 \text{ mEq}}{50 \text{ mEq}}$$

$$X = 25 \text{ ml}$$

You should administer 25 ml of sodium bicarbonate solution.

Potassium puzzle

The doctor prescribes 30 mEq of potassium chloride oral solution for your patient. The solution contains 60 mEq in every 15 ml. How many milliliters of solution should you give the patient? This is how to solve this problem.

- Set up a proportion using X as the unknown quantity:

$$\frac{X}{30 \text{ mEq}} = \frac{15 \text{ ml}}{60 \text{ mEq}}$$

- Cross-multiply the fractions:

$$X \times 60 \text{ mEq} = 15 \text{ ml} \times 30 \text{ mEq}$$

- Find X by dividing both sides of the equation by 60 mEq and canceling units that appear in both the numerator and denominator:

$$\frac{X \times 60 \text{ mEq}}{60 \text{ mEq}} = \frac{15 \text{ ml} \times 30 \text{ mEq}}{60 \text{ mEq}}$$

$$X = 7.5 \text{ ml}$$

You should administer 7.5 ml of oral potassium chloride solution.

Now you're cooking! Keep up the good work!

Frequently used conversions

In clinical practice, a doctor may write a medication order in one measurement system, but the medication may be available in a different system. For example, he might order 10 gr of a drug that's available only in milligrams.

To convert medication orders from one system to another, you must know the equivalent measures. If you have trouble remembering the most frequently used equivalents, jot the equivalents on an index card, laminate the card, and tuck it in your pocket for easy reference.

A conversion excursion

Two conversions that are frequently used, especially in adult and pediatric intensive care units, are pounds (lb) to kilograms (kg) and inches (") to centimeters (cm). These conversions are used to determine body weight and body surface.

Making these conversions isn't hard if you remember the general rules:
• Remember that 1 kg equals 2.2 lb. To convert pounds into kilograms, just divide the number of pounds by 2.2. To convert kilograms to pounds, multiply the number of kilograms by 2.2.
• Remember that 1" equals 2.54 cm. To convert inches to centimeters, just multiply the number of inches by 2.54. To convert centimeters to inches, divide the number of centimeters by 2.54.

Equivalent measure conversions

The following examples show how to do equivalent measure conversions.

You say pounds, I say kilograms

To prepare medications for your hypotensive patient, you must determine her weight in kilograms. You know that she weighs 125 lb, but how much is this in kilograms? This is how to find out.
• You know that 1 kg equals 2.2 lb. So set up a proportion using X as the unknown weight:

$$\frac{X}{125 \text{ lb}} = \frac{1 \text{ kg}}{2.2 \text{ lb}}$$

• Cross-multiply the fractions:

$$X \times 2.2 \text{ lb} = 1 \text{ kg} \times 125 \text{ lb}$$

• Find X by dividing both sides of the equation by 2.2 lb and canceling units that appear in both the numerator and denominator:

$$\frac{X \times 2.2 \text{ lb}}{2.2 \text{ lb}} = \frac{1 \text{ kg} \times 125 \text{ lb}}{2.2 \text{ lb}}$$

$$X = 56.8 \text{ kg}$$

Your patient weighs 56.8 kg.

You say milliliters, I say cups

A patient who's on a clear liquid diet must drink 480 ml of water for lunch. How many cups is this equal to? This is how to find out:
• You know that 1 cup equals 240 ml. So set up a proportion using X as the unknown number:

$$\frac{X}{480 \text{ ml}} = \frac{1 \text{ cup}}{240 \text{ ml}}$$

• Cross-multiply the fractions:

$$X \times 240 \text{ ml} = 1 \text{ cup} \times 480 \text{ ml}$$

• Find X by dividing both sides of the equation by 240 ml and canceling units that appear in both the numerator and denominator:

$$\frac{X \times 240 \text{ ml}}{240 \text{ ml}} = \frac{1 \text{ cup} \times 480 \text{ ml}}{240 \text{ ml}}$$

$$X = 2 \text{ cups}$$

Your patient needs to drink 2 cups of water.

Wow! I can convert anything!

You say tablespoons, I say milliliters

The doctor orders 30 ml of milk of magnesia for your patient's heartburn. How many tablespoons is this? This is how to find out.
• You know that 1 tbs contains 15 ml, so set up a proportion using X as the unknown number:

$$\frac{X}{30 \text{ ml}} = \frac{1 \text{ tbs}}{15 \text{ ml}}$$

• Cross-multiply the fractions:

$$X \times 15 \text{ ml} = 1 \text{ tbs} \times 30 \text{ ml}$$

• Find X by dividing both sides of the equation by 15 ml and canceling units that appear in both the numerator and denominator:

$$\frac{X \times 15 \text{ ml}}{15 \text{ ml}} = \frac{1 \text{ tbs} \times 30 \text{ ml}}{15 \text{ ml}}$$

$$X = 2 \text{ tbs}$$

Your patient needs 2 tbs of milk of magnesia.

Quick quiz

1. The Arabic numeral 575 in Roman numerals is:
   A.   DXXXXXXXV.
   B.   DLXXV.
   C.   CCCCCLXXV.

Answer: B. To convert 575, break it into its component parts (500, 70, and 5); then translate the parts into Roman numerals.

2. The symbol ss represents:
   A.   one-half.
   B.   the abbreviation for "without."
   C.   the dram symbol.

Answer: A. The symbol ss represents one-half in Roman numerals.

3. Drugs that are measured in units include:
   A.   penicillin V, insulin, and heparin.
   B.   co-trimoxazole.
   C.   cough medicine.

Answer: A. Penicillin V, insulin, and heparin are measured in units.

4. Electrolytes are measured in:
   A.   grains.
   B.   milligrams.
   C.   milliequivalents.

Answer: C. Most electrolytes, such as potassium chloride, are measured in milliequivalents.

5. When converting pounds to kilograms you should:
   A   multiply by 2.54.
   B.   divide by 2.2.
   C.   divide by 2.54.

Answer: B. One kilogram equals 2.2 lb. By dividing pounds by 2.2, you obtain kilograms.

6. Before the metric system was established, doctors and pharmacists used the:
   A.   apothecaries' system.
   B.   avoirdupois system.
   C.   household system.

Answer: A. Used before the metric system, the apothecaries' system is being phased out today.

7. The equivalent in milliliters of 55 U of NPH insulin (U-100) is:
   A.   55 ml.
   B.   0.55 ml.
   C.   5 ml.

Answer: B. To do the conversion, set up the proportion:

$$\frac{X}{55\ U} = \frac{1\ ml}{100\ U}$$

Cross-multiply the fractions; then divide both sides of the equation by 100 U and cancel units that appear in both the numerator and denominator to get 0.55 ml:

$$\frac{X \times \cancel{100\ U}}{\cancel{100\ U}} = \frac{1\ ml \times 55\ \cancel{U}}{100\ \cancel{U}}$$

$$X = 0.55\ ml$$

8. The equivalent of 1 tsp of medication in milliliters is:
   A.   15 or 16 ml.
   B.   4 or 5 ml.
   C.   30 or 32 ml.

Answer: B. 1 tsp equals 4 or 5 ml.

Scoring

☆☆☆ If you answered all eight items correctly, fantastic! Reward yourself with a minim of ice cream (all right, you can have a pint!).

☆☆ If you answered five to seven items correctly, good job! Have a fluidram of champagne (enjoy every minim!).

☆ If you answered fewer than five items correctly, keep at it. In the meantime, have a dram of chocolate (savor every grain!).

Part III

Recording drug administration

7   **Drug orders**   109

8   **Administration records**   121

Drug orders

Just the facts

In this chapter, you'll learn:

♦ what a drug order consists of

♦ how to interpret drug orders using standard abbreviations

♦ how to use military time

♦ how to avoid making drug administration errors

♦ what to do about unclear drug orders.

A look at drug orders

Administering drugs is one of your most critical nursing responsibilities. It's also the area with the smallest margin for error. How can you prevent drug errors? The best way is by knowing how to read and correctly interpret drug orders. To do this, you need to understand what a drug order is and how it's used.

Direct handoff

In an outpatient setting, a doctor or health care professional who's licensed to prescribe drugs writes an order on a prescription form and gives it directly to the patient.

Keyboard, form, or fax

The routine for prescribing drugs is different in inpatient facilities. There, a doctor generates a drug order in one of the following ways:

• by entering the order into a computer system that transmits it to the pharmacy and to the nurses' station

• by writing the order on the drug order sheet in the patient's chart

• by faxing the order to a pharmacy (this method saves time by preventing an order from staying in a patient's chart or computer until the chart or computer is checked; however, the patient's confidentiality may be breached by this method).

What's in a drug order?

The drug order sheet in a patient's chart must include all patient information, so it's usually stamped with the patient's admission data plate. When writing the order, the doctor includes:

- date and time of the order
- name of the drug, either generic or trade
- dosage form in metric, apothecaries', or household measurement
- abbreviation for the route of administration, such as P.O., I.M., S.C., I.V., P.R., P.V., or S.L. (in some health care facilities, if the route isn't specified, the staff may assume that the oral route is preferred)
- administration schedule written as times per day or as number of hours between doses
- restrictions or specifications related to the order
- doctor's signature or name and code number in a computerized system (one signature or name and code number is sufficient after a group of orders)
- doctor's registration number for controlled drugs, if applicable.

Following orders

Standard guidelines exist for writing drug orders. Being aware of these guidelines will help you interpret drug orders:

- The generic name of a drug is written entirely in lowercase letters.
- The trade or brand name of a drug begins with a capital letter.
- Drug abbreviations are written entirely in capital letters; however, drug names usually aren't abbreviated.
- Write information in this sequence: drug name, dose, administration route, and time and frequency of administration.

A brief look at abbreviating

Standard abbreviations are used to describe drug measurements, dosages, routes and times of administration, and related terms. The Joint Commission on Accreditation of Healthcare Organizations requires every health care facility to develop a list of approved abbreviations for staff use. (See *Making it short and sweet.*)

Remember that abbreviations can be easily misinterpreted, especially if they're written carelessly or quickly. If an abbreviation seems unusual or doesn't make sense to you, contact the doctor for clarification. Then clearly write the correct term in your revision and transcription.

Making it short and sweet

Standard abbreviations are handy for quick and accurate transcription of medication orders and documentation of drug administration. Use these abbreviations for drug measurements, dosage forms, routes and times of administration, and related terms.

Drug and solution measurements

cc	cubic centimeter
fl dr	fluidram
fl oz	fluidounce
g	gram
gal	gallon
gr	grain
gtt	drop
kg	kilogram
L	liter
mcg	microgram
ml	milliliter

Drug dosage forms

cap	capsule
DS	double strength
elix	elixir
LA	long-acting
liq	liquid
SA	sustained action
SR	sustained release
Sol	solution
Susp tab	suspension tablet

Routes of drug administration

A.D.	right ear
A.S.	left ear
A.U.	each ear
I.M.	intramuscular
I.V.	intravenous
NG tube	nasogastric tube
O.D.	right eye

(continued)

Making it short and sweet *(continued)*

Routes of drug administration *(continued)*

O.S.	left eye
O.U.	each eye
P.O. or p.o.	by mouth
P.R.	rectally
P.V.	vaginally
S.C.	subcutaneous
S.L.	sublingually

Times of drug administration

a.c.	before meals
b.i.d.	twice a day
h.s.	at bedtime
p.c.	after meals
p.r.n.	as needed
q.a.m.	every morning
q.d.	every day
q.o.d.	every other day
q4h	every 4 hours
stat	immediately

Miscellaneous abbreviations

AMA	against medical advice
ASAP	as soon as possible
BP	blood pressure
BPM	breaths (or beats) per minute
$\bar{c}$	with
D/C or dc	discontinue
KVO	keep vein open
MR	may repeat
NKA	no known allergies
NPO	nothing by mouth
P	pulse
R	respiration
<	less than
>	greater than
$\bar{s}$	without

Military time

Study the two clocks below to better understand military time. The clock on the left represents the hours from 1 a.m. (0100 hours) to noon (1200 hours). The clock on the right represents the hours from 1 p.m. (1300 hours) to midnight (2400 hours).

Marching in time (military time, that is)

Some doctors and health care facilities require pharmacologic orders and medication administration records to be written and transcribed in military time. For example, an order might read *Lasix 40 mg I.V. b.i.d. at 0900 and 2100 hours.* (See *Military time.*)

Simply confusing or confusingly simple?

Military time might seem confusing at first, but it's actually simple to use. This method of time is based on a 24-hour system. Here's how it works:
• To write single-digit times from 1:00 a.m. to 12:59 p.m., put a zero before the times and remove the colon. For example, 1:00 a.m. is written 0100 hours.
• To write double-digit times from 1:00 a.m. to 12:59 p.m., just remove the colon. For example, 11:00 a.m. becomes 1100 hours.
• The minutes after the hour remain the same. For example, 4:45 a.m. becomes 0445 hours.
• To write times from 1:00 p.m. to 12 midnight, simply add 1200 to the hour and remove the colon. For example, 1:00 p.m. becomes 1300 hours (1:00 + 12:00); 3:30 p.m. becomes 1530 hours (3:30 + 12:00); and 12:00 a.m (midnight) becomes 2400 hours (12:00 + 12:00).

Step to it! Learn military time.

• To write the minutes between 12:01 a.m. and 12:59 a.m., start over with zero. For example, 12:33 a.m. becomes 0033 hours.

Dealing with drug orders

Once you determine that a drug order contains all the necessary information, you can begin to interpret it. Read on to find guidelines for dealing with illegible handwriting, timing drug administration, renewing drug orders, and discontinued drug orders. (See *Say it in English.*)

Hospital hieroglyphics

If any required information is missing or if the doctor's handwriting is illegible, check with the doctor and clarify the order before signing the transcription. Also ask the doctor for clarification if nonstandard abbreviations are used.

Once the order is clear, sign it and send a copy to the pharmacy where the drug will be dispensed according to your facility's policy.

Calibrating the clinical clock

Although the drug order sheet tells you when to give a drug, the actual administration time depends on three things:
• your facility's policy (for drugs that are given a specific number of times per day)
• the nature of the drug
• the drug's onset and duration of action.

Be sure to administer drugs within a half hour of the times specified on the drug order sheet.

After giving a drug, record the actual time of administration on the medication administration record.

Reevaluate, renew, reorder

Health care facilities also have policies for how often drug orders must be renewed. For example, narcotics may need to be re-ordered every 24, 48, or 72 hours. This allows health care professionals to reevaluate the patient's need for the drug and to adjust the dosage or frequency of administration, if necessary.

Remember that I.V. fluids — such as normal saline solution, dextrose and water, and total parenteral nutrition solutions — are considered drugs. Check all I.V. fluid orders carefully. Most health care facilities provide guidelines for the renewal of I.V. fluids as well as for other drugs.

Cheat sheet

Administering drugs

• Give within 30 minutes of the specified time.
• Record actual administration time.
• If discontinued, make sure the doctor writes a new order.
• With each order, ensure that the appropriate drug is being administered.

Say it in English

The following examples illustrate how to read and interpret a wide range of drug orders.

Drug order	Interpretation
Colace 100 mg P.O. b.i.d. p.c.	Give 100 mg of Colace by mouth twice a day after meals.
Vistaril 25 mg I.M. q3h p.r.n.	Give 25 mg of Vistaril intramuscularly every 3 hours as needed.
Increase Duramorph to 6 mg I.V. q8h	Increase Duramorph to 6 mg intravenously every 8 hours.
folic acid 1 mg P.O. q.d.	Give 1 mg of folic acid by mouth daily.
Minipress 4 mg P.O. q6h, hold for sys BP < 120	Give 4 mg of Minipress by mouth every 6 hours; withhold the drug if the systolic blood pressure falls below 120 mm Hg.
nifedipine 30 mg S.L. q4h	Give 30 mg of nifedipine sublingually every 4 hours.
Begin aspirin 325 mg P.O. q.d.	Begin giving 325 mg of aspirin by mouth daily.
Persantine 75 mg P.O. t.i.d.	Give 75 mg of Persantine by mouth three times a day.
aspirin grains v P.O. t.i.d.	Give 5 grains of aspirin by mouth three times a day.
Vasotec 2.5 mg P.O. q.d.	Give 2.5 mg of Vasotec by mouth daily.
1,000 ml D_5W c̄ KCl 20 mEq I.V. at 100 ml/h	Give 1,000 ml of dextrose 5% in water with 20 milliequivalents of potassium chloride intravenously at a rate of 100 milliliters per hour.
D/C penicillin I.V., start penicillin G 800,000 U P.O. q6h	Discontinue intravenous penicillin; start 800,000 units of penicillin G by mouth every 6 hours.
diphenhydramine 25–50 mg P.O. h.s. p.r.n.	Give 25 to 50 mg of diphenhydramine by mouth at bedtime as needed.

Short-winded — Persantine 75 mg P.O. t.i.d.

Give 75 mg of Persantine by mouth three times a day. — Long-winded

Stop! That's an order.

If the doctor decides to discontinue a drug before the original order runs out, he must write a new order. These orders also must be precise.

For example, if an order reads *D/C K* and the patient is receiving vitamin K and potassium chloride, you'll need to contact the doctor to clarify which medication he wants to discontinue.

Handling ambiguous drug orders

All too often, drug orders are unclear because of nonstandard abbreviations, illegible handwriting, incorrect dosages, or missing information. It helps if handwritten orders are neat, with drugs spelled correctly. (See *Don't struggle with difficult orders.*)

Rule #1: Bad input equals bad output.

Even if the doctor enters drug orders into the computer system, your interpretation skills are still extremely important. Although computers solve the problem of illegible handwriting, they can't correct human error. A computer will accept the wrong drug, the wrong dose, the wrong route, and the wrong frequency. It's up to you to verify the input.

Rule #2: Advocate appropriate administration.

Your responsibility in interpreting orders includes making sure that the ordered drug is an appropriate treatment. This is where your role as patient advocate comes in. To make sure the drug you're asked to administer is appropriate:
• Think critically; don't be timid about asking for clarification and justification.
• Know the action of each drug you give and the purpose for which it's given.
• If a drug order seems questionable, use all available resources to check it. For example, ask the doctor, the pharmacist, and your colleagues and refer to a drug handbook.
• Always check the five "rights" before giving a drug. (See *Right on target*, page 118.)
• Check and recheck all your drug calculations.
• Never administer a drug that's improperly labeled or that you personally didn't draw from a vial.
• Never use open or unmarked I.V. solution bags.

All this goes for I.V. fluids too!

Practice with poorly written orders

The following are examples of poorly written drug orders that need to be clarified by the doctor who wrote them. See if you can find the errors.

What?

K 40 mEq I.V. q.d. — It's unclear what drug is being ordered. Is it vitamin K or potassium chloride (KCl)? If it's KCl, remember that this electrolyte must be diluted in I.V. fluid before administration.

Computers aren't perfect. They won't correct an incorrect order. It's up to you!

Before you give that drug!

Don't struggle with difficult orders

The combination of poor handwriting and inappropriate abbreviations on a drug order can lead to confusion and medication errors. Ask the doctor to clarify an order that's difficult to understand or one that seems wrong.

		FREEDOM HOSPITAL		DOCTOR'S ORDERS

FREEDOM HOSPITAL

UNIT NO. 4 SOUTH, 432 A
NAME JOE JACKSON
ADDRESS 33 SHORT STREET
CITY HOPE, NJ BIRTH 2·21·24

DOCTOR'S ORDERS
INSTRUCTIONS
1. Each time a physicians writes a medication order, detach top copy and send to pharmacy.
2. Rule off unused lines after last copy (Pink) has been sent to pharmacy.

DO NOT USE THIS SHEET UNLESS A NUMBER SHOWS. 1

DATE	TIME	ORDERS	DOCTOR'S SIGNATURE	NURSE'S SIGNATURE
2/14/0	12³⁰ p			
				O. Alexander
6/29/01				
6/30/01				

Discharge diagnoses in order of decreasing priority must be supplied at time of patient's discharge.

If you can't read something on the drug order, ask the doctor for clarification.

Advice from the experts

Right on target

No matter how careful you are when administering drugs, occasional errors can still occur. The pharmacy may even send the wrong drug. To avoid errors and keep your patient safe, never administer a drug without first checking off the "five rights" at your patient's bedside.

Right drug

Right dose

Right route

Right time

Right patient

I think you're right.

How?

Digoxin 0.25 mg q.d. — The administration route is missing. Digoxin may be given orally as a pill or elixir or may be given I.V.

When?

Nifedipine 10 mg P.O. — The frequency of administration is missing. Nifedipine can be given in a single dose for hypertension, or it can be given on another schedule as a maintenance drug. In the latter case, it's usually given orally.

Quick quiz

1. Drug abbreviations should be written:
    A.   in lowercase letters.
    B.   in capital letters.
    C.   with the first letter in capitals.

Answer: B. Drug abbreviations should be avoided but, when they're used, they should be written in all capital letters.

2. The correct abbreviation for "after meals" is:
   A.   P.O.
   B.   P.R.
   C.   p.c.

Answer: C. P.O. stands for "by mouth," and P.R. stands for "by rectum."

3. The abbreviation MR stands for:
   A.   milligram.
   B.   may repeat.
   C.   may remove.

Answer: B. Milligram is abbreviated mg, and "may remove" has no standard abbreviation.

4. The order *morphine 4 mg I.M. q4h p.r.n. pain, hold for respiratory rate < 12 BPM* means:
   A.   Give morphine 4 mg intramuscularly four times a day for pain; hold for respiratory rate less than 12 breaths per minute.
   B.   Give morphine 4 mg intramuscularly every 4 hours for pain; hold for respiratory rate greater than 12 breaths per minute.
   C.   Give morphine 4 mg intramuscularly every 4 hours as needed for pain; hold for respiratory rate less than 12 breaths per minute.

Answer: C. "Every 4 hours" is abbreviated q4h, the abbreviation p.r.n. means "as needed," and the symbol < means "less than."

5. In military time, 3:08 p.m. is:
   A.   0308 hours.
   B.   1508 hours.
   C.   1308 hours.

Answer: B. To convert a time from 1:00 p.m. to 12 midnight, remove the colon and add the number to 1200 hours.

6. "Give Dilantin 150 mg by mouth twice a day at 0900 hours and 2100 hours; draw Dilantin levels every other day" can be written on a drug order as:
   A.   *Dilantin 150 mg P.O. b.i.d at 9:00 a.m. and 9:00 p.m., draw Dilantin levels q.o.d.*
   B.   *Dilantin 150 mg P.O. t.i.d. at 9:00 a.m. and 9:00 p.m., draw Dilantin levels q.d.*
   C.   *Dilantin 150 mp I.V. b.i.d. at 9:00 a.m. and 9:00 p.m., draw Dilantin levels q.o.d.*

Answer: A. In answer B, t.i.d. means "three times a day," and q.d. means "every day." In answer C, mp isn't a standard abbreviation, and I.V. means "intravenously."

7. Using a computer to order drugs:
   A.   decreases patient confidentiality.
   B.   helps pinpoint errors in writing orders.
   C.   solves the problem of illegible handwriting.

Answer: C. A computer can make orders legible, but it can't spot errors.

8. The five "rights" of drug administration are:
   A.   drug, dose, route, time, and patient.
   B.   drug, filter, solution, doctor, and shift.
   C.   drug, order, signature, time, and patient.

Answer: A. To help ensure patient safety, go through this checklist before administering a drug.

Scoring

☆☆☆ If you answered all eight items correctly, wow! You're error-free!

☆☆ If you answered five to seven correctly, you're almost there! You can spot an incorrect order, recognize standard abbreviations, and read hospital hieroglyphics!

☆ If you answered fewer than five correctly, keep going! You're acquiring the art of the drug order!

Administration records

Just the facts

In this chapter, you'll learn:

♦ what types of medication administration record systems are used

♦ how to document on the administration record

♦ how to prevent drug errors

♦ how to report drug errors.

A look at administration records

Maintaining accurate medication administration records is a vital nursing responsibility, both for legal reasons and for patient safety. The liability risk of the health care provider may increase if medication administration isn't properly documented. Documentation that's missing or inaccurate can lead to drug errors that can jeopardize your patient's health.

Record-keeping systems

Three main types of medication administration record systems are used today: the Kardex, the medication administration record (MAR), and computer charting.

The Kardex system

The Kardex system consists of a set of large index cards in a hinged file. The file is usually kept in the medication room or on the medication cart, although individual cards also may be clipped to the patient's chart or clipboard.

The MAR

Another widely used system, the MAR is an $8\frac{1}{3}'' \times 11''$ form that goes into the patient's chart. It also may be kept in the medication room on the medication cart in a three-ring binder or may be clipped to the patient's chart or clipboard while the patient is hospitalized. On discharge, the MAR is placed in the patient's chart. (Some units use a combination of the Kardex and the MAR.)

Computer charting

A third system, computer charting, is being used increasingly by more health care facilities. Information is entered into a computer that automatically generates a list of administration times for all scheduled medications. Computer systems cut the risk of drug errors caused by illegible handwriting. (See *Record keeping in the computer age.*)

Record keeping in the computer age

As health care facilities purchase or develop computer systems, manufacturers offer increased choices among medication monitoring programs.

From simple...
Computerized record systems range from simple to sophisticated. In the simplest systems, the computer is used as a word processor or typewriter.

...to sophisticated
In more sophisticated systems, doctors can order drugs from the pharmacy by typing the drug's name, or they can select specific drugs by searching through various listings, such as pharmacologic categories, pharmacokinetic categories, and disease-related uses.

The computer indicates whether the pharmacy has the drug. The order then goes into the pharmacy's computer for filling. The order also generates the patient's record, on which the nurse can document medication administration.

Benefits bit by bit
Computer systems offer the following advantages:
• When drug orders are changed, the pharmacy receives immediate notification, so drugs arrive on the unit faster.
• The pharmacy's computer can immediately confirm or deny a drug's availability.
• Nurses can document on medication administration records quickly and easily.
• Nurses can see at a glance which drugs have been administered and which still need to be given.
• Errors from misinterpreted handwriting are eliminated.
• Records can be stored on disk in addition to, or instead of, paper copies.

Chart smart

Different forms, same info

The medication Kardex below illustrates the kind of information required on all types of medication administration forms. Although different facilities may use different forms, virtually all require the patient information, date, drug information, time of administration, and the nurse's initials after administering the drug.

INITIAL	SIGNATURE	INITIAL	SIGNATURE
SA	Sally Adams RN		
JJ	Joan Johnson RN		

R = REFUSED O = OMITTED F = FASTING

JOE JACKSON
33 SHORT STREET
HOPE N.J 2·21·24
UNIT : 4 SOUTH 432 A

ALLERGIES
NKA

DATE ORD.	STOP DATE	MEDICATION DOSE ROUTE FREQUENCY	R.N. INT.	HR.	2/14	2/15	2/16	2/17	2/18	2/19
2/14	2/18	carbidopa/levodopa (SINEMET) 25/250 P.O. Q.I.D	SA	A 10	X					
				P 2						
				P 6						
				P 10						
2/14	2/19	benztropine mesy-late (COGENTIN) 1.0 mg P.O. T.I.D.	SA	A 10	X					
				P 2						
				P 6						
2/14	2/16	diphenhydramine hydrochloride (BENADRYL) 25 mg. P.O. H.S.	SA	P 10						

ROUTINE MEDICATIONS
FREEDOM HOSPITAL
DIAGNOSIS & SURGERY   AGE   SEX   PHYSICIAN   ROOM   NAME

My ruling: Keep good records!

See you in court

No matter what type of medication charting system your facility uses, you must still record certain standard information. Standardization allows medication administration records to be used as legal documents if it ever becomes necessary to prove that a drug dose was given. (See *Different forms, same info*.)

Documentation

In general, documentation reflects the tasks, assessments, and procedures nurses perform. Documenting on the administration record indicates that you've carried out the doctor's order.

Does that say subcutaneous or subcuticular?

Before transcribing the doctor's orders, make sure that they're complete, clear, and correct. If you detect a problem, contact the doctor before sending the order to the pharmacy. If you detect a problem after the order goes to the pharmacy, contact both the doctor and the pharmacy.

Is that 1 mg I.V. over 10 minutes or 10 mg over 1 minute?

Information recorded on a Kardex or MAR must be written legibly in ink. All handwritten or computerized administration records must contain patient information, drug information, and signatures. *Remember:* Transcribing drug orders requires close attention because even a small discrepancy can cause a major drug error.

Recording patient information

If your facility uses a computerized system, you don't need to transcribe patient information onto the administration record. It's already there because the admissions office enters the patient information into the system, and the pharmacy adds information, such as the patient's height, weight, and allergies.

If you use a Kardex or MAR, stamp the form with the patient's admission data plate. If this isn't available, copy the information from the patient's identification bracelet.

Identification, please

Record the patient's full name, hospital identification number, unit number, bed assignment, and allergies, even those that aren't drug related. If the patient doesn't have any known allergies, write "NKA."

If the name of his insurance carrier is written on his identification bracelet, record this, too. *Transcribe the information exactly as it appears on the bracelet.*

Recording drug information

Next, transcribe from the doctor's order complete information about every drug the patient is taking. Include dates and drug names, dosages, strengths, dosage forms, administration routes, and administration times.

It's a date!

You must always record these dates on the administration record: the date the prescription was written; the date the drug should begin, if this is different from the original order date; and the date the drug should be discontinued.

At some facilities, the time and date the drug should begin are recorded together. This serves as a reference for the time to discontinue a drug when a limited period is indicated. Many facilities also have a standard length of time a drug may be given before it's automatically discontinued.

Full name, please

Record the drug's full generic name. If the doctor ordered the drug using a proprietary name, record this name as well. Don't use abbreviations, chemical symbols, research names, or special facility names. This can cause medication errors or delay therapy.

Working on your strength

When recording drug strength, be sure to write the actual amount of the drug to be administered. If the dose you administer varies in any way from the strength or amount ordered, note this in a special area on the administration record, if there is one, or in the patient's progress notes.

For example, document whether the patient refused to take a drug, consumed only part of a drug, or vomited shortly after taking a drug.

As a matter of form...

Also record the drug dosage form that the doctor ordered. Then decide whether the form is appropriate, considering the patient's special needs.

For example, if sustained-action theophylline tablets are ordered for a patient with a nasogastric tube, he won't be able to take the tablets orally. You'll have to crush them before administering them through the tube.

However, crushing sustained-action tablets destroys the drug's integrity and alters its therapeutic action. So, you'll need to contact the doctor and discuss an alternative drug dosage form.

Be sure to record the dosage form.

Tracking the route

Recording the route of administration is especially critical for drugs that may be given by two different routes. For example, acetaminophen can be given orally or rectally. Other drugs can be given by only one correct route; for example, NPH insulin may be given subcutaneously but not intravenously.

If you administer a drug by a different route than that which the doctor originally ordered, indicate that change, along with the reason and authorization for the change.

Citing the site

When administering a drug by a parenteral route, record the injection site to facilitate site rotation. Most administration forms include a numbered list of recognized sites, allowing you to record the site by its number.

Schedule scheme

The doctor's order should include an administration schedule, such as t.i.d. or q6h. Transcribe the schedule onto the administration record; then convert it into actual times based on your facility's policy and the drug's availability, characteristics, onset, and duration of action.

For example, t.i.d. may mean 9 a.m., 1 p.m., and 5 p.m. in one facility and 10 a.m., 2 p.m., and 6 p.m. in another. Similarly, b.i.d. may be 10 a.m. and 6 p.m. or 10 a.m. and 10 p.m.

Working around the clock

Remember that time notations are based on a 24-hour clock, unless otherwise specified. This means that the hour appearing first on a 24-hour clock should appear first in the time notation.

In other words, if an administration schedule is 2-10-2-10, the first 2 represents 2 a.m., or 0200 hours; the first 10 represents 10 a.m., or 1000 hours; the second 2 is 2 p.m., or 1400 hours; and the second 10 is 10 p.m., or 2200 hours.

Under special circumstances

Some facilities have separate administration records or specially designated areas of the regular administration record for recording single orders or special drug orders. Special orders include drugs given p.r.n., large-volume parenteral drugs, and dermatologic and ophthalmic medications dispensed in bottles or tubes.

Other facilities put single orders or special drugs on the regular administration record. If this is the case where you work, be careful to distinguish these drugs from those that are regularly scheduled. All facilities have special forms for recording controlled substances. (See *Controlling controlled substances*.)

Cheat sheet

Administering drugs

- If parenteral, record the injection site.
- Immediately document the times of all administrations.
- If unscheduled, record the exact time.
- If given late or not at all, document the reasons.
- Always sign any documentation on the administration record.

Chart smart

Controlling controlled substances

Federal and state laws regulate the dispensation, administration, and documentation of controlled substances. When these substances are issued to a unit, they're accompanied by a perpetual inventory record, often called a "narcotics record" or "controlled inventory record."

A paper trail

If the doctor orders a controlled substance for your patient, document its administration on the administration record and the perpetual inventory record. When you remove a dose from the locked storage site, note this information on the perpetual inventory record:
- date and time the dose is removed
- amount of the drug remaining in the locked storage site
- patient's full name
- doctor's name
- drug dose
- your signature.

   If you have to discard any of the dose, have another nurse verify the amount discarded and ask her to sign the form, too.

A nurse really has to keep track of her time!

Time is of the essence

Immediately after giving a drug, document the time of administration to keep you from mistakenly giving the drug again. For scheduled drugs, you'll usually initial the appropriate time slot for the date that the drug is administered.

Scheduled drugs are considered on time if they're given within a half hour of the ordered time. For unscheduled drugs, such as single doses and p.r.n. drugs, record the exact time of administration in the appropriate slot.

If you don't give a drug on time or if you miss a dose, document the reason on either the administration record or the patient's progress notes. Facility policy may require you to initial and circle the particular time missed on the administration record to draw attention to it.

Your signature here

Every time you document on the administration record, you must sign it. First, initial the record after transcribing from the doctor's order sheet. Many facilities also require the nurse to perform a chart check and initial the doctor's order sheet on a line after the last order. This indicates that all orders have been transcribed correctly onto the administration record.

If someone other than a nurse transcribes the order, a nurse must co-sign the order sheet and the administration record.

Initiate initialing

You also need to sign the administration record after giving a drug. Put your initials in the appropriate space on the form. Make sure that they're legible and always sign them the same way. If another nurse on your unit has the same initials or name, use your middle initial to avoid confusion.

In addition, write your full name, title, and initials in the signature section of the administration record. This information must appear on every record you initial when administering drugs.

Assuring quality and preventing errors

Each facility has its own method for tracking errors in drug administration. Unfortunately, many errors aren't documented because the administering nurses are afraid to report them. But tracking and documenting errors allows the performance improvement team to recommend ways to prevent them in the future and keep patients safe.

Eradicating errors

One way to decrease medication errors is by adhering to your facility's policies, suggested safety precautions, and performance improvement recommendations. Another way is by transcribing orders carefully from the doctor's order sheet to the administration record.

Sensible safeguards

To avoid transcription errors, follow these guidelines:
• Transcribe orders in a quiet area where you can concentrate without interruptions.
• Before signing the order sheet and initialing the administration record, carefully check both forms.
• Follow your facility's policy for reviewing orders. Some require nurses to check all patient charts for new orders several times each shift and check orders written within the past 24 hours. Other facilities give one shift, usually the night shift, this last responsibility.

Before you give that drug!

Conquering confusion

Before giving a drug, remind yourself of these essential tactics.

Remember the rights.
Check off the five "rights" — right drug, right dose, right route, right time, and right patient.

Look at the label.
Examine drug labels closely — many of them look alike.

Notice the name.
Pay attention! Many drugs have similar-sounding names. Consider the examples below:
• Compazine and Thorazine
• hydromorphone and morphine
• Pavulon and Parafon
• cefoxitin and Ceftin.

Refusing to give a drug

On rare occasions, you may be asked to administer a drug about which you feel uncomfortable. You can legally refuse to administer a drug under these circumstances:
• if you think the dosage prescribed is too high
• if you think the drug might interact dangerously with other drugs the patient is taking or substances such as alcohol
• if you think the patient's physical condition contraindicates use of the drug.

The right way to say no

When you refuse to carry out a drug order, be sure to:
• Notify your immediate supervisor so she can make alternative arrangements (such as assign a new nurse or clarify the order).
• Notify the prescribing doctor if your supervisor hasn't done so.
• If your employer requires it, document that the drug wasn't given and explain why.

Keeping a cool head

Many drug errors occur because nurses are in a hurry or are unfamiliar with a drug. Try to take your time. Remember that many drugs are derivatives of other drugs, so they have similar names. If a drug is new to you, use available resources to find out all you can about it. (See *Conquering confusion*, page 129.)

Reporting drug errors

Even though you take precautions, you may still make a drug error. Or you may administer a drug correctly only to have a patient react negatively to it. When this happens, the value of meticulous documentation becomes clear.

The right response

If you make an error, follow these steps:
• Notify the doctor immediately.
• Consult the pharmacist. He can provide information about drug interactions, solutions to dose-related problems such as what to do about an overdose or an omitted dose, and an antidote, if needed.
• Continue to assess the patient, paying close attention to the drug's action and possible effects.
• Follow your facility's policy for documenting drug errors. You may have to complete an incident report for legal purposes. If so, clearly document what happened without defending an action or placing blame. Record the names and functions of everyone involved and what actions they took to protect the patient after the error was discovered.

Cheat sheet

In case of error

• Notify the doctor.
• Consult the pharmacist.
• Assess the patient throughout.
• Follow the proper drug error documentation policy.

Quick quiz

1.   You may be required to circle and initial the time slot of a medication if:
    A.   you missed the dose or gave it late.
    B.   the administration time has changed.
    C.   another nurse forgot to administer a drug.

Answer: A. Circling and initialing the time slot signals to the next nurse that the dose was missed or late. The nurse then refers to the single-order or p.r.n. section of the MAR to find the actual administration time. That way, she doesn't mistakenly administer the next dose too soon.

2. The information on the patient's admission data plate should include his:

    A. full name, social security number, birth date, and doctor's name.

    B. full name, hospital identification number, bed location, unit number, and allergies.

    C. full name, address, and doctor's name.

Answer: B. The patient's address and insurance company name also may appear on the plate.

3. Injection site rotation is facilitated when each nurse documents:

    A. time of the last injection.

    B. date of the last injection.

    C. site of the last injection.

Answer: C. Recording the site tells the next nurse what sites have already been used so she doesn't use them again.

4. You have the right to refuse to administer a drug if:

    A. you don't trust the doctor.

    B. you think the dosage is too high.

    C. it doesn't arrive on time to give it on schedule.

Answer: B. You can also refuse to administer a drug if it would interact dangerously with other drugs the patient is taking or if it's contraindicated for his physical condition.

5. When a computerized system is used, the admissions office enters patient information and the pharmacy adds:

    A. care plan changes.

    B. allergy alerts.

    C. perpetual records.

Answer: B. The pharmacy also adds other information, such as the patient's height and weight.

6. To avoid confusion, nurses with the same initials should sign the administration record with:

    A. their identification numbers.

    B. pens with different colors of ink.

    C. their middle initials.

Answer: C. Also be sure to write legibly and always sign the same way.

7. You should transcribe orders:
   A. in the patient's room.
   B. at the nurses' station.
   C. in a quiet area.

Answer: C. Transcribing in a quiet area without distractions will help you concentrate.

8. Immediately after you administer a drug, you should:
   A. document its effectiveness.
   B. document the time of administration.
   C. order the next dose of the drug from the pharmacy.

Answer: B. Documenting the time of administration immediately after you give the drug keeps you from mistakenly giving the drug again.

Scoring

☆☆☆ If you answered all eight items correctly, amazing! You've been voted best nurse at the Administration Academy Awards!

☆☆ If you answered six or seven correctly, fantastic! Here's your Oscar for best supporting nurse!

☆ If you answered less than six correctly, keep your chin up! You're still a record setter!

Part IV

Oral, topical, and rectal drugs

9 Calculating oral drug dosages 135

10 Calculating topical and rectal drug dosages 163

Calculating oral drug dosages

Just the facts

In this chapter, you'll learn:

♦ how to read drug labels to obtain accurate information for calculations

♦ how to administer drugs safely

♦ how to calculate oral dosages of tablets, capsules, and liquids

♦ how to calculate dosages using different measurement systems.

A look at oral drugs

Drugs that are administered by the oral route are usually in tablet, capsule, or liquid form. Most oral drugs are available in a limited number of strengths or concentrations. Therefore, your ability to calculate prescribed dosages for various drug forms and strengths is an important skill.

Reading oral drug labels

Before you can administer an oral drug safely, you must make sure that it's the correct drug and the correct dosage. Your first step is to read the label carefully, noting the drug's name, dose strength, and expiration date.

Drug name

When reading a drug label, check the generic name first. If the drug has two names, the generic name usually appears in smaller print. The generic name is the accepted nonproprietary name, which is a simplified form of the drug's chemical name.

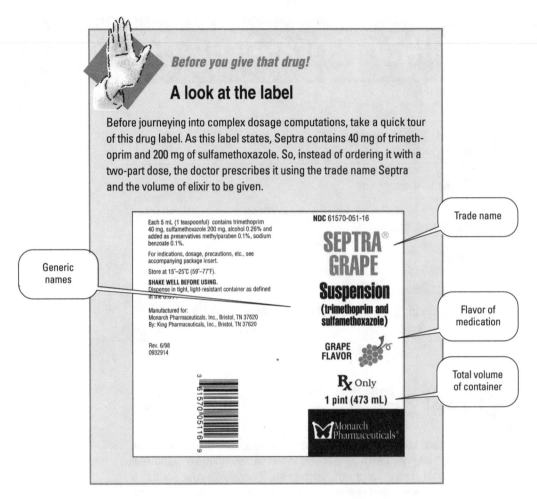

Before you give that drug!

A look at the label

Before journeying into complex dosage computations, take a quick tour of this drug label. As this label states, Septra contains 40 mg of trimethoprim and 200 mg of sulfamethoxazole. So, instead of ordering it with a two-part dose, the doctor prescribes it using the trade name Septra and the volume of elixir to be given.

Generic names

Trade name

Flavor of medication

Total volume of container

Each 5 mL (1 teaspoonful) contains trimethoprim 40 mg, sulfamethoxazole 200 mg, alcohol 0.26% and added as preservatives methylparaben 0.1%, sodium benzoate 0.1%.

For indications, dosage, precautions, etc., see accompanying package insert.

Store at 15°–25°C (59°–77°F).

SHAKE WELL BEFORE USING.
Dispense in tight, light-resistant container as defined in the U.S.P.

Manufactured for:
Monarch Pharmaceuticals, Inc., Bristol, TN 37620
By: King Pharmaceuticals, Inc., Bristol, TN 37620

Rev. 6/98
0932914

NDC 61570-051-16

SEPTRA® GRAPE

Suspension
(trimethoprim and sulfamethoxazole)

GRAPE FLAVOR

Rx Only

1 pint (473 mL)

Monarch Pharmaceuticals®

Next, note the drug's trade name, also called the brand or proprietary name. This name, given by the manufacturer, usually appears first on the label, followed by the registration symbol.

Two in one

Some oral medications actually contain two drugs. The labels for these combination drugs list both generic names and their doses. These drugs are ordered by the trade name and the number of capsules or tablets or the volume of elixir to be given — for example, *Septra 1 tsp q12hr.* (See *A look at the label.*)

The name game

A drug may have several trade names, but it has only one generic name. For example, the generic drug diazepam goes by the trade names Valium, Valrelease, and Zetran.

However, some drugs are so widely used and so well known by their generic names that the manufacturer never gives them a trade name. One example is atropine sulfate.

Meeting the standard

The initials U.S.P. or N.F. may appear after the drug name. They stand for two legally recognized standards for drugs: United States Pharmacopeia and National Formulary. These initials mean

Before you give that drug!

Look-alike labels: Tablets and capsules

Don't let yourself be fooled by look-alike labels. The names on the following tablet and capsule labels are examples of look-alikes and sound-alikes that you must read carefully to avoid medication errors.

Norpramin and Norpace
On first glance, you may be easily confused by these medication names, which could lead to a medication error that could harm the patient. Norpramin is a tricyclic antidepressant, whereas Norpace is an antiarrhythmic. Inadvertent substitution of the anti-depressant Norpramin for Norpace wouldn't control the patient's arrhythmia and could lead to serious complications.

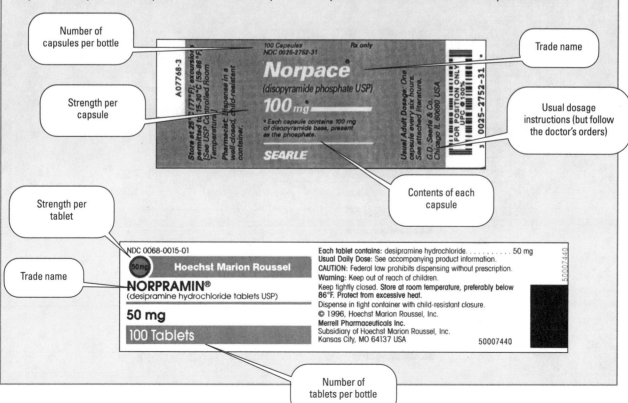

that a drug has met standards of purity, potency, and storage, which are enforced by the Food and Drug Administration.

Dose strength

After checking the drug name, look for the dose strength on the label. Pay close attention: The labels and containers for different concentrations of the same drug may look exactly alike except for the listing of the drug's concentration. (See *Look-alike labels: Tablets and capsules*, page 137.)

> Knowing the strength of a drug is important. Pay attention!

Before you give that drug!

Look-alike labels: Oral solutions

The oral solution labels below are examples of look-alikes that you're likely to encounter. Reading labels carefully can help you avoid medication errors.

> This one is Augmentin 200 mg/5 ml.

> The label reads 400 mg/5 ml of Augmentin—two times the concentration of the other one.

Oral examination

The same is true for oral solutions. The labels can look similar for different concentrations of the same drug. Be sure to examine the label closely. (See *Look-alike labels: Oral solutions.*)

Expiration date

Finally, check the expiration date. This vital information is often overlooked. Expired drugs may be chemically unstable and may no longer provide the correct dose. If a drug has expired, return it to the pharmacy so that it can be disposed of properly and the patient can be reimbursed.

Administering oral drugs safely

The first rule in assuring the safest possible administration of drugs is to triple-check drug labels and drug orders. Safe drug administration requires you to compare the doctor's order as transcribed on the medication administration record against the drug label *three times*. (See *Say it three times: Check orders and labels*, page 140.)

Proceed with caution

The doctor has ordered *150 mg ranitidine (Zantac) P.O. b.i.d.* for your patient. Before giving the drug, follow this procedure to the letter:

Open the patient's medication drawer, find the drug labeled ranitidine (Zantac) 150 mg, and note that it's in oral tablet form.

Place the labeled drug next to the transcribed order on the administration record and carefully compare each part of the label to the order.

If the drug is supplied in bulk or in a stock bottle, transfer one tablet from the supply to a medication container, pouring from the supply to the lid and then into the container without handling the tablet.

Before returning the supply to the drawer or shelf, once again compare the label to the order on the administration record, and note whether this is the right administration time. *Once you've removed a drug from its container, you can't ever be certain that it's the correct drug unless you've carefully compared the label to the administration record while pouring.*

Now, go to the patient's bedside, check his identification bracelet, and do your third drug check, comparing the label to the order and checking the administration time again. Then give the drug.

If the drug comes in a unit-dose packet, don't remove it from the packet until you're at the patient's bedside and ready to administer it. Then do your third drug check. Remove the drug from the packet and give it to the patient, using the packet label for comparison when recording your administration information. (See *Unit-dose packaging*.)

Discovering discrepancies

If you notice discrepancies between the administration record and the drug label, check them out. For example, suppose the adminis-

Before you give that drug!

Say it three times: Check orders and labels

The secret of drug safety is to check, check, and check again. Before giving a drug, carefully compare the drug's label with each part of the medication administration record, holding the label next to the administration record to ensure accuracy. The example below walks you through the steps for administering *furosemide (Lasix) 40 mg P.O.*

Check drug names.
• Read the drug's generic name on the administration record and compare it to the generic name on the label. They both should say *furosemide.*
• Read the trade name on the administration record and compare it to the trade name on the label. They both should say *Lasix.*

Check the dosage, route, and record.
• Read the dose on the administration record and compare it to the dose on the label. They both should say *40 mg.*
• Read the route specified on the administration record and note the dose form on the label. The record should say *P.O.,* and the label should say *oral tablet.*

• Note any special considerations on the administration record, such as "aspiration precautions (head of bed elevated to 45 degrees for all P.O. intake)," "Patient is HOH (hard of hearing)," or "Patient is blind."

Check orders and labels three times.
Follow this routine three times before giving the drug. Do it the first time when you obtain the drug from floor stock or the patient's supply. Do it the second time before placing the drug in the medication cup or other administration device. Finally, do it the third time before replacing the stock drug bottle on the shelf or removing the drug from the unit-dose package at the patient's bedside.

Unit-dose packaging

Tablets or capsules in unit doses may be dispensed on a card with the drugs sealed in bubbles or in strips with each drug separated by a tear line. Unit doses of liquids may be packaged in small sealed cups with identifying information on the cover.

Save time with the unit-dose system

Using the unit-dose drug distribution system gives you more time for evaluating patient responses to drugs and for teaching patients about their drug regimens.

More exact (that's a fact)

This timesaving system provides the exact dose of medication needed for each patient. The pharmacist computes the number of tablets or the volume of liquid and prepares the proper dose for administration. Errors are decreased because the drug remains in its labeled container until you give it to the patient.

Don't throw away your calculator yet.

Does this mean your dosage calculation days are over? Not by a long shot. Some facilities don't use the unit-dose system, and others have systems that don't operate 24 hours a day. So your dosage calculation skills are still vitally important.

tration record specifies Ceclor and the drug packet is labeled cefaclor. Check your drug handbook and you'll find that Ceclor is a trade name for cefaclor.

Or, suppose the drug packet is labeled Ceclor 250 mg and the dose on the administration record is 500 mg. In this case, you need to calculate the required dose. Scrupulous attention to details like these will help ensure safe, error-free drug administration.

Unit-dose systems

Many facilities use the unit-dose system, which provides prepackaged drugs in single-dose containers and decreases the need for dosage calculations. (See *Save time with the unit-dose system.*)

Calculating dosages

Despite the prevalence of unit-dose systems, calculations are still necessary in many patient situations. For example, you may have to determine individualized dosages for special patients. You also must know how to convert between measurement systems to determine how many tablets, capsules, or other dosage forms to administer. (See *Special delivery drug dosages*.)

You'll often use ratios and fractions in proportions to calculate drug dosages and to convert between measurement systems. The following section reviews these mathematical concepts and shows step-by-step calculations. (See *Helpful hints to minimize math mistakes*.)

Using ratios, fractions, and proportions

Ratios and fractions are two ways to express the numerical relationship between things. A proportion expresses equality between two ratios or fractions. Proportions may be written using ratios, as in

$$1 : 3 :: 2 : 6$$

Advice from the experts

Special delivery drug dosages

Even if your facility uses the unit-dose system, you'll still need to calculate dosages for some patients. For example, patients on critical care units, pediatric patients, and geriatric patients require individualized medication dosages that may be unusually large or small.

The nearest milligram
Some patients need dosages that are calculated to the nearest milligram instead of the nearest 10 mg. For them, the correct calculation of the exact dosage can mean the difference between an underdose and an overdose. A few examples of drugs that are measured to the nearest milligram or microgram are digoxin, levothyroxine sodium, and many pediatric drugs.

Changing the delivery route
Some people can't handle drugs that are delivered by the usual route because their ability to absorb, distribute, metabolize, or excrete drugs is impaired. Some patients can't absorb drugs from the GI tract because of upper GI disorders or surgery; defi-

ciencies of gastric, pancreatic, or intestinal secretions; or passive congestion of GI blood vessels from severe heart failure. These patients need drugs in parenteral form in larger-than-average oral doses. Smaller doses of a drug can be used when the drug is given I.V. because the drug may be delivered to the bloodstream more efficiently and is more readily absorbed.

Don't forget these special patients
Other patients who need individualized dosages include those with conditions that cause abnormal drug distribution from the GI tract or from parenteral sites to the sites of action. Premature infants and patients with low serum protein levels or severe liver or kidney disease who can't metabolize or excrete drugs as readily as normal patients also require special drug dosages. You can help individualize drug regimens for these patients by assessing their kidney or liver function, monitoring blood levels of drugs, and calculating exact dosages.

or using fractions, as in

$$\frac{1}{3} = \frac{2}{6}$$

When proportions are expressed using ratios, the product of the means (the inside numbers), equals the product of the extremes (the outside numbers):

$$\overset{\text{means}}{\overbrace{2:4::1:2}}$$
$$\underset{\text{extremes}}{\underbrace{2:4::1:2}}$$

so,

$$4 \times 1 = 2 \times 2$$

When proportions are expressed as fractions, their cross products are equal:

$$\frac{3}{6} \bowtie \frac{6}{12}$$

so,

$$3 \times 12 = 6 \times 6$$

Equally mean and extreme

When a proportion is expressed using ratios, the units of the mean on one side of the equal sign must match the units of the extreme on the other side, and vice versa:

mg : tablet :: mg : tablet

When a proportion is expressed using fractions, the units of measure in the numerators must be the same, and the units of measure in the denominators must be the same:

$$\frac{\text{mg}}{\text{tablet}} = \frac{\text{mg}}{\text{tablet}}$$

Denominators are the same.

Numerators are the same.

Four rules for calculating drug dosages

To help you prevent calculation and medication errors and to simplify your calculations, remember these four rules.

Use correct units of measure

Using the incorrect unit of measure is one of the most common dosage calculation errors. When calculating doses, matching units of measure in the numerator and denominator cancel each other, leaving the correct unit of measure in the answer. Here's an example:

How many milligrams of a drug are in two tablets if one tablet contains 5 mg of the drug?

☝ State the problem as a proportion:

$$5 \text{ mg} : 1 \text{ tablet} :: X : 2 \text{ tablets}$$

✌ Remember that the product of the means equals the product of the extremes:

> **Multiply the means.**

$$1 \text{ tablet} \times X = 5 \text{ mg} \times 2 \text{ tablets}$$

> **Multiply the extremes.**

👌 Solve for X. Divide each side of the equation by the known value, 1 tablet, and cancel units that appear in both the numerator and denominator:

$$\frac{1 \text{ tablet} \times X}{1 \text{ tablet}} = \frac{5 \text{ mg} \times 2 \text{ tablets}}{1 \text{ tablet}}$$

$$X = 10 \text{ mg}$$

Double-check decimals and zeros

An error in the number of decimal places or zeros in a dosage calculation can cause a tenfold or greater dose error. Here's an example using both decimals and zeros: The doctor orders *0.05 mg Synthroid P.O.*, but the only Synthroid on hand is in tablets that contain 0.025 mg each. How many tablets should you give?

• State the problem as a proportion:

$$0.025 \text{ mg} : 1 \text{ tablet} :: 0.05 \text{ mg} : X$$

• The product of the means equals the product of the extremes:

$$1 \text{ tablet} \times 0.05 \text{ mg} = 0.025 \text{ mg} \times X$$

• Solve for X by dividing each side of the equation by 0.025 mg and canceling units that appear in both the numerator and denominator, carefully checking decimal placement:

$$\frac{1 \text{ tablet} \times 0.05 \text{ mg}}{0.025 \text{ mg}} = \frac{0.025 \text{ mg} \times X}{0.025 \text{ mg}}$$

$$X = 2 \text{ tablets}$$

Question strange answers

Be especially careful to recheck suspicious-looking calculations. For example, if a dosage calculation suggests giving 25 tablets or 200 ml of suspension, assume that you've made an error and check your figures. If you're still unsure about your results, have another nurse check your calculation.

Get out the calculator

A handheld calculator can improve the accuracy and speed of your calculations, *but it can't guarantee accuracy*. You still must set up proportions carefully and double-check units of measure and decimal places.

> **Cheat sheet**
>
> **Calculation key**
> • Use correct units of measure.
> • Double-check units of measure and decimal places.
> • Check answers that seem wrong.
> • Use a calculator.

Special considerations

Occasionally when administering oral drugs, you may come across unusual situations that require you to take a few extra steps.

Divided doses

Most tablets, capsules, and similar dose forms are available in only a few strengths. Usually, you'll administer one tablet or one-half of a scored tablet.

Breaking an unscored tablet in portions smaller than one-half usually creates inaccurate doses. If a dose smaller than one-half of a scored tablet or any portion of an unscored tablet is needed, you should substitute a commercially available solution or suspension or have one prepared by the pharmacist.

You can also ask the pharmacist to crush the tablet and measure an exact dose. However, some oral preparations shouldn't be opened, broken, scored, or crushed because those actions change the drug's effect. (See *Be cautious with tablets and capsules,* page 146.)

> Don't leave half-dosages to chance. Be exact!

All things being equianalgesic

At times, you may need to convert a dose of an analgesic from the parenteral route to the oral route. If so, equianalgesic charts provide the information you need to recalculate the dose necessary to produce the desired pain control. These charts use morphine sulfate as the gold standard for comparing pain control. (See *Equianalgesic charts: A painless path for converting dosages,* page 147.)

Be cautious with tablets and capsules

Before you break or crush a tablet or capsule, call the pharmacist to see if the drug is available in smaller dosage strengths or in liquid form for patients who have difficulty swallowing. Also check your drug handbook — or check with the pharmacist — to see if altering the drug will affect its action. Drugs that shouldn't be altered include the following:

• sustained-release drugs, also called extended-release, timed-release, or controlled-release

• capsules that contain tiny beads of medication, although you may empty the contents of some of these capsules into a beverage, pudding, or applesauce

• enteric-coated tablets, which have a hard coating — usually shiny or glossy — that's designed to protect the upper GI tract from irritation

• buccal and sublingual tablets.

Tips for crushing and breaking
If you need to crush a tablet, use a chewable form, which is softer. The easiest method is to crush the tablet while it's still in its package, using a hemostat or pill crusher. Or you can remove it from the package and crush it with a mortar and pestle.

If you need to break a tablet, use one that's scored. Carefully cut the tablet on the score line with a scalpel or a pill cutter. Enlist the pharmacist's help when you need to break a tablet into smaller pieces than the score allows or when you must administer a portion of a capsule. If you need to break an unscored tablet, have the pharmacist crush, weigh, and dispense it in two equal doses.

Real world problems

When calculating the number of tablets to administer, use proportions. Set up the first ratio or fraction with the known tablet strength. Set up the second ratio or fraction with the prescribed dose and the unknown quantity of tablets or capsules. Then solve for X to determine the correct dose. To illustrate, here are some typical patient situations.

The acetaminophen answer

The doctor orders *650 mg acetaminophen P.O. STAT* for your patient, but the drug is available only in 325-mg tablets. How many tablets should you give?

Here's the calculation using ratios.

• Set up the first ratio with the known tablet strength:

325 mg : 1 tablet

• Set up the second ratio with the desired dose and the unknown number of tablets:

650 mg : X

the Real World

Equianalgesic charts: A painless path for converting dosages

When substituting one analgesic for another, equianalgesic charts provide the information you need to calculate the dose necessary to produce the desired pain control (equianalgesic effect).

These charts use morphine sulfate as the *gold standard* for comparison. On most charts, doses for a variety of drugs are listed; each dose provides pain relief equivalent to 10 mg of I.M. morphine. Here's an example of an equianalgesic chart.

Medication	I.M. dose	P.O. dose
Morphine	10 mg	30 mg
Codeine	1.5 mg	7.5 mg
Hydromorphone	2 mg	4 mg
Levorphanol	130 mg	200 mg
Meperidine	75 mg	300 mg

Remember: Every dose on the equianalgesic chart provides an equivalent amount of pain control, and any change in medication requires a doctor's order.

• Put these ratios into a proportion:

$$325 \text{ mg} : 1 \text{ tablet} :: 650 \text{ mg} : X$$

• Set up the equation by multiplying the means and the extremes:

$$1 \text{ tablet} \times 650 \text{ mg} = 325 \text{ mg} \times X$$

• Solve for X by dividing both sides of the equation by 325 mg and canceling units that appear in both the numerator and denominator:

$$\frac{1 \text{ tablet} \times 650 \text{ mg}}{325 \text{ mg}} = \frac{325 \text{ mg} \times X}{325 \text{ mg}}$$

$$X = 2 \text{ tablets}$$

The clozapine clue

Your patient is prescribed *250 mg clozapine P.O. daily.* How many tablets should he take if each tablet contains 100 mg?

Here's the calculation using ratios.

- Set up the first ratio with the known tablet strength:

$$100 \text{ mg} : 1 \text{ tablet}$$

- Set up the second ratio with the desired dose and the unknown number of tablets:

$$250 \text{ mg} : X$$

- Put these ratios into a proportion:

$$100 \text{ mg} : 1 \text{ tablet} :: 250 \text{ mg} : X$$

- Multiply the means and the extremes:

$$1 \text{ tablet} \times 250 \text{ mg} = 100 \text{ mg} \times X$$

- Divide each side of the equation by 100 mg and cancel units that appear in both the numerator and denominator:

$$\frac{1 \text{ tablet} \times 250 \text{ \cancel{mg}}}{100 \text{ \cancel{mg}}} = \frac{100 \text{ \cancel{mg}} \times X}{100 \text{ \cancel{mg}}}$$

$$X = 2\frac{1}{2} \text{ tablets}$$

Gliding through glyburide

The doctor's order reads *glyburide 1.5 mg iii tablets P.O. daily.* What is the total dose in milligrams?

Here's the solution using fractions.

- Set up the first fraction with the known tablet strength:

$$\frac{1.5 \text{ mg}}{1 \text{ tablet}}$$

- Set up the second fraction with the desired dose and the unknown number of milligrams:

$$\frac{X}{3 \text{ tablets}}$$

- Put these fractions into a proportion:

$$\frac{X}{3 \text{ tablets}} = \frac{1.5 \text{ mg}}{1 \text{ tablet}}$$

- Cross-multiply the fractions:

$$X \times 1 \text{ tablet} = 1.5 \text{ mg} \times 3 \text{ tablets}$$

• Divide both sides of the equation by 1 tablet and cancel units that appear in both the numerator and denominator:

$$\frac{X \times 1\,\text{tablet}}{1\,\text{tablet}} = \frac{3\,\text{tablets} \times 1.5\,\text{mg}}{1\,\text{tablet}}$$

$$X = 4.5\,\text{mg}$$

The answer is 4.5 mg.

Calculating liquid dosages

In addition to administering tablets to your patients, you'll also give them liquid medications in suspension or elixir form. Before calculating a dose, read the label carefully to identify the dosage strength in a specified amount of solution. Then check the label for the expiration date.

More real world problems

In each of the following problems, use the proportion method to calculate the amount of solution. Set up the first ratio or fraction with the known solution strength, and set up the second ratio or fraction with the desired dose and the unknown quantity. Then solve for X to find the correct dose.

Here are some typical patient situations.

the Real World

Pay attention to the suspension.

Your patient is receiving 500 mg of Ceclor oral suspension. The label says Ceclor 250 mg/5 ml, and the bottle contains 100 ml. How many milliliters of Ceclor should you give?

Here's the solution using fractions.

• Set up the first fraction with the known solution strength:

$$\frac{5\,\text{ml}}{250\,\text{mg}}$$

• Set up the second fraction with the desired dose and the unknown number of milliliters:

$$\frac{X}{500\,\text{mg}}$$

- Put these fractions into a proportion:

$$\frac{X}{500 \text{ mg}} = \frac{5 \text{ ml}}{250 \text{ mg}}$$

- Cross-multiply the fractions:

$$X \times 250 \text{ mg} = 5 \text{ ml} \times 500 \text{ mg}$$

- Solve for X by dividing both sides of the equation by 250 mg and canceling units that appear in both the numerator and denominator:

$$\frac{X \times 250 \text{ mg}}{250 \text{ mg}} = \frac{5 \text{ ml} \times 500 \text{ mg}}{250 \text{ mg}}$$

$$X = \frac{2,500 \text{ ml}}{250}$$

$$X = 10 \text{ ml}$$

Erythromycin enigma

Your patient needs 400 mg of erythromycin oral suspension. The label says erythromycin 200 mg/5 ml. How many milliliters should you give?

Here's the calculation using ratios

- Set up the first ratio with the unknown solution strength:

$$X : 400 \text{ mg}$$

- Set up the second ratio with the desired dose and the known number of milliliters:

$$5 \text{ ml} : 200 \text{ mg}$$

- Put these ratios into a proportion:

$$X : 400 \text{ mg} :: 5 \text{ ml} : 200 \text{ mg}$$

- Set up an equation by multiplying the extremes and the means:

$$X \times 200 \text{ mg} = 5 \text{ ml} \times 400 \text{ mg}$$

- Solve for X by dividing both sides of the equation by 200 mg and canceling units that appear in both the numerator and denominator:

$$\frac{X \times 200 \text{ mg}}{200 \text{ mg}} = \frac{5 \text{ ml} \times 400 \text{ mg}}{200 \text{ mg}}$$

$$X = \frac{2,000 \text{ ml}}{200}$$

$$X = 10 \text{ ml}$$

Don't dally over Dilantin doses.

The doctor orders *100 mg Dilantin oral suspension t.i.d.* for your patient. The label says Dilantin 125 mg/5 ml. How many milliliters should you give?

Here's the calculation using ratios.

• Set up the first fraction with the unknown solution strength:

$$X : 100 \text{ mg}$$

• Set up the second fraction with the desired dose and the known number of milligrams:

$$5 \text{ ml} : 125 \text{ mg}$$

• Put these fractions into a proportion:

$$X : 100 \text{ mg} :: 5 \text{ ml} : 125 \text{ mg}$$

• Set up an equation by multiplying the means and the extremes:

$$100 \text{ mg} \times 5 \text{ ml} = 125 \text{ mg} \times X$$

• Solve for X by dividing each side of the equation by 125 mg and canceling units that appear in both the numerator and denominator:

$$\frac{100 \cancel{\text{ mg}} \times 5 \text{ ml}}{125 \cancel{\text{ mg}}} = \frac{125 \cancel{\text{ mg}} \times X}{125 \cancel{\text{ mg}}}$$

$$\frac{500 \text{ ml}}{125} = X$$

$$X = 4 \text{ ml}$$

Diluting powders

Some drugs become unstable when they're stored as liquids, so they're supplied in powder form. Before giving these drugs, dilute them with the appropriate diluent, usually tap water. Read the drug labels carefully to see how much diluent to add.

After adding the diluent, read the labels again to determine the dose strengths contained in the volumes of fluid. To calculate the dosages, use the ratio and proportion method.

Weighing in

The dose concentration in oral solutions is expressed as the weight — or dose strength — of the drug contained in a volume of solution. For example, Lasix oral solution is provided as 10 mg/ml. So the solution contains 10 mg of Lasix (drug weight) in 1 ml (solution volume).

Measuring oral solutions

To administer an oral solution accurately, measure it with a medicine cup, dropper, or syringe. Medicine cups are calibrated to measure solutions in milliliters, tablespoons, teaspoons, drams, and ounces. For accuracy, hold the cup at eye level while pouring the solution.

For good measure

Drugs that are prescribed in drops usually are packaged with a dropper. If they are not, use a standard dropper. They can be used to measure solutions in milliliters or teaspoons. After measuring and administering a drug from a multiple-dose container, store it as directed on the drug label.

Don't use syringes to administer oral drugs — if you leave the plastic tip on by mistake, the patient can swallow or aspirate it.

Two-step dosage calculations

Most dosage calculations require more than one equation. For example, the doctor may order a drug in grains, but it may be available only in tablet, capsule, or liquid form in milligrams. When this happens, you need to convert from one measurement system to another before deciding how much medication to administer. (See *When you need a new measure.*)

Keeping in step

When converting between measurement systems, first consult a conversion table to find the standard equivalent value — the equivalent between the two measurement systems. Then use the ratio and proportion method to calculate the correct dose. Put the standard equivalent values in the first ratio or fraction and put the quantity ordered and the unknown quantity in the second ratio or fraction.

Still more real world problems

The examples below show how to convert from one measurement system to another and then how to calculate the correct dose.

Wary of apothecaries' units?

Your patient's order, written in apothecaries' units, reads *aspirin gr x P.O. daily*, but the unit-dose package says *aspirin 325 mg*. How many tablets should you administer daily?

Here's how to solve this using fractions.

• Recall that in apothecaries' units, "aspirin gr x" indicates 10 gr of aspirin. Refer to *Measure for measure*, page 98, to find that 1 gr is equivalent to approximately 60 mg. Then set up the first fraction with the standard equivalent values:

$$\frac{60 \text{ mg}}{1 \text{ grain}}$$

• Set up the second fraction with the unknown quantity in the appropriate position:

$$\frac{X}{10 \text{ grains}}$$

• Put these fractions into a proportion:

$$\frac{60 \text{ mg}}{1 \text{ grain}} = \frac{X}{10 \text{ grains}}$$

• Cross-multiply the fractions to set up an equation:

$$60 \text{ mg} \times 10 \text{ grains} = X \times 1 \text{ grain}$$

• Solve for X by dividing both sides of the equation by 1 gr and canceling units that appear in both the numerator and denominator:

$$\frac{60 \text{ mg} \times 10 \cancel{\text{ grains}}}{1 \cancel{\text{ grain}}} = \frac{X \times 1 \cancel{\text{ grain}}}{1 \cancel{\text{ grain}}}$$

$$X = 600 \text{ mg}$$

• The dose to be given is 600 mg. Now determine the number of tablets to give by setting up a proportion:

$$\frac{X}{600 \text{ mg}} = \frac{1 \text{ tablet}}{325 \text{ mg}}$$

Advice from the experts

When you need a new measure

To easily determine a dose when you must first convert to a different system of measurement, remember these tips:

• Read the drug order thoroughly, paying close attention to decimal places and zeros.

• Convert the dose from the system in which it's ordered to the system in which it's available.

• Calculate the number of capsules or tablets or the amount of solution needed to obtain the desired dose.

Keeping in step with the two-step calculations?

- Cross-multiply the fractions:

$$X \times 325 \text{ mg} = 1 \text{ tablet} \times 600 \text{ mg}$$

- Solve for X by dividing each side of the equation by 325 mg and canceling units that appear in both the numerator and denominator:

$$\frac{X \times 325 \text{ mg}}{325 \text{ mg}} = \frac{1 \text{ tablet} \times 600 \text{ mg}}{325 \text{ mg}}$$

$$X = \frac{600 \text{ tablets}}{325}$$

$$X = 1\tfrac{4}{5} \text{ tablets}$$

- Because giving 1⅘ tablets would be very difficult, round off the dose to 2 tablets.

Pondering a prescription

A prescription reads *phenobarbital gr ¼ take gr ½ t.i.d. P.O. daily.* How many milligrams of phenobarbital should this patient receive?

Here's how to solve this using fractions.

- Convert "gr ¼" to milligrams by consulting a conversion table such as that in *Measure for measure,* page 98. You'll see that 1 gr equals approximately 60 mg.
- Set up the first fraction with the standard equivalent values:

$$\frac{60 \text{ mg}}{1 \text{ grain}}$$

- Set up the second fraction with the unknown quantity in the appropriate position:

$$\frac{X}{\text{grain } \tfrac{1}{4}}$$

- Put these fractions into an equation:

$$\frac{60 \text{ mg}}{1 \text{ grain}} = \frac{X}{\text{grain } \tfrac{1}{4}}$$

- Cross-multiply the fractions:

$$60 \text{ mg} \times \text{grain } \tfrac{1}{4} = X \times 1 \text{ grain}$$

• Solve for X by dividing each side of the equation by 1 gr and canceling units that appear in both the numerator and denominator:

$$\frac{X \times 1 \cancel{grain}}{1 \cancel{grain}} = \frac{60 \text{ mg} \times \cancel{grain} \, \frac{1}{4}}{1 \cancel{grain}}$$

$$X = 60 \text{ mg} \times \frac{1}{4}$$

$$X = 15 \text{ mg}$$

• Now we know that grain ¼ equals 15 mg. However, the prescribed dose is grain ½. Calculate the number of milligrams to give the patient by setting up a proportion:

$$\frac{X}{\text{grain } \frac{1}{2}} = \frac{15 \text{ mg}}{\text{grain } \frac{1}{4}}$$

• Cross-multiply the fractions:

$$X \times \text{grain } \frac{1}{4} = 15 \text{ mg} \times \text{grain } \frac{1}{2}$$

• Solve for X by dividing both sides of the equation by grain ¼ and canceling units that appear in both the numerator and denominator:

$$\frac{X \times \cancel{\text{grain } \frac{1}{4}}}{\cancel{\text{grain } \frac{1}{4}}} = \frac{15 \text{ mg} \times \cancel{\text{grain } \frac{1}{2}}}{\cancel{\text{grain } \frac{1}{4}}}$$

$$X = \frac{15 \text{ mg} \times \frac{1}{2}}{\frac{1}{4}}$$

$$X = \frac{7 \, \frac{1}{2} \text{ mg}}{\frac{1}{4}}$$

$$X = 30 \text{ mg}$$

The dose to be given is 30 mg.

Digoxin dilemma

Your patient receives a prescription for 62.5 mcg of digoxin elixir P.O. daily. The elixir label reads 0.05 mg/ml. How many milliliters of digoxin should you give?

Here's how to solve this using ratios.
• Convert micrograms to milligrams. Recall that 1,000 mcg equals 1 mg.
• Set up the first ratio with this standard equivalent value:

1 mg : 1,000 mcg

- Set up the second ratio with the unknown quantity in the appropriate position:

$$X : 62.5 \text{ mcg}$$

- Put these ratios into a proportion:

$$1 \text{ mg} : 1{,}000 \text{ mcg} :: X : 62.5 \text{ mcg}$$

- Multiply the means and the extremes:

$$X \times 1{,}000 \text{ mcg} = 1 \text{ mg} \times 62.5 \text{ mcg}$$

- Solve for X by dividing both sides of the equation by 1,000 mcg and canceling units that appear in both the numerator and denominator:

$$\frac{X \times 1{,}000 \text{ mcg}}{1{,}000 \text{ mcg}} = \frac{1 \text{ mg} \times 62.5 \text{ mcg}}{1{,}000 \text{ mcg}}$$

$$X = \frac{62.5 \text{ mg}}{1{,}000}$$

$$X = 0.0625 \text{ mg}$$

- The prescribed dose is 62.5 mcg, or 0.0625 mg. Calculate the number of milliliters to be given by setting up a proportion:

$$0.0625 \text{ mg} : X :: 0.05 \text{ mg} : 1 \text{ ml}$$

- Set up an equation by multiplying the means and the extremes:

$$X \times 0.05 \text{ mg} = 1 \text{ ml} \times 0.0625 \text{ mg}$$

- Solve for X by dividing each side of the equation by 0.05 mg and canceling the units of measure that appear in both the numerator and denominator:

$$\frac{X \times 0.05 \text{ mg}}{0.05 \text{ mg}} = \frac{1 \text{ ml} \times 0.0625 \text{ mg}}{0.05 \text{ mg}}$$

$$X = 1.25 \text{ ml}$$

The dose to be given is 1.25 ml.

I knew I should have paid more attention in math class!!!

The desired-over-have method

The desired-over-have method is another way to solve two-step problems. This method uses fractions to express the known and unknown quantities in proportions:

$$\frac{\text{amount desired}}{\text{amount you have}} = \frac{\text{equivalent amount desired}}{\text{equivalent amount you have}}$$

Make sure the units of measure used in the numerator and denominator of the first fraction correspond to the units of measure in the numerator and denominator of the second fraction.

The following three problems show how to use the desired-over-have method.

The potassium chloride puzzler

The doctor orders *60 mEq potassium chloride liquid* as a one-time dose, but the only solution on hand contains 20 mEq/15 ml. How many tablespoons should you give the patient?

Here's the calculation.

• Convert milliliters to tablespoons by consulting a conversion table such as that in *Measure for measure*, page 98. You'll see that 15 ml equals 1 tbs. Therefore, 20 mEq of the solution on hand equals 1 tbs.

• Set up the first fraction with the amount desired over the amount you have:

$$\frac{60 \text{ mEq}}{20 \text{ mEq}}$$

• Set up the second fraction with the unknown amount desired — represented by X — in the appropriate position:

$$\frac{X}{1 \text{ tbs}}$$

• Put these fractions into a proportion:

$$\frac{X \text{ desired}}{1 \text{ tbs have}} = \frac{60 \text{ mEq desired}}{20 \text{ mEq have}}$$

• Cross-multiply the fractions:

$$X \times 20 \text{ mEq} = 1 \text{ tbs} \times 60 \text{ mEq}$$

• Solve for X by dividing each side of the equation by 20 mEq and canceling units that appear in both the numerator and denominator:

$$\frac{X \times 20 \cancel{\text{ mEq}}}{20 \cancel{\text{ mEq}}} = \frac{1 \text{ tbs} \times 60 \cancel{\text{ mEq}}}{20 \cancel{\text{ mEq}}}$$

$$X = 3 \text{ tbs}$$

The patient should receive 3 tbs of potassium chloride liquid.

Cheat sheet

The desired-over-have method

• The amount desired over the amount you have equals the equivalent amount desired over the equivalent amount you have.

• For both fractions, verify that the units of measure correspond for the numerator and denominator.

Acetaminophen alley

The order reads *acetaminophen elixir 650 mg P.O. stat.* The pharmacy sends you Tylenol 325 mg/5 ml. How many teaspoons do you give?

Here's the calculation.

• Convert milliliters to teaspoons by consulting a conversion table such as that in *Measure for measure*, page 98. You'll see that 1 tsp equals 5 ml.

• Set up the first fraction with the amount desired over the amount you have:

$$\frac{650 \text{ mg}}{325 \text{ mg}}$$

• Set up the second fraction with the unknown amount desired in the appropriate position:

$$\frac{X}{1 \text{ tsp}}$$

• Put these fractions into a proportion:

$$\frac{X}{1 \text{ tsp have}} = \frac{650 \text{ mg desired}}{325 \text{ mg have}}$$

• Cross-multiply the fractions:

$$X \times 325 \text{ mg} = 1 \text{ tsp} \times 650 \text{ mg}$$

• Solve for X by dividing both sides of the equation by 325 mg and canceling units that appear in both the numerator and denominator:

$$\frac{X \times \cancel{325 \text{ mg}}}{325 \text{ mg}} = \frac{1 \text{ tsp} \times 650 \cancel{\text{ mg}}}{325 \cancel{\text{ mg}}}$$

$$X = 2 \text{ tsp}$$

The patient should receive 2 tsp of acetaminophen elixir.

Teaspoon teaser

The doctor orders *60 mg phenobarbital elixir at h.s. daily* for your patient, but the drug is available only as 20 mg/5 ml. How many teaspoons should you give?

Here's the calculation.

• Convert milliliters to teaspoons by consulting a conversion chart. You'll see that 1 tsp equals 5 ml.

• Set up the first fraction with the amount desired over the amount you have:

$$\frac{60 \text{ mg}}{20 \text{ mg}}$$

• Set up the second fraction with the unknown amount desired in the appropriate position:

$$\frac{X}{1 \text{ tsp}}$$

• Put these fractions into a proportion:

$$\frac{60 \text{ mg}}{20 \text{ mg}} = \frac{X}{1 \text{ tsp}}$$

• Cross-multiply the fractions:

$$60 \text{ mg} \times 1 \text{ tsp} = 20 \text{ mg} \times X$$

• Solve for X by dividing both sides of the equation by 20 mg and canceling units that appear in both the numerator and denominator:

$$\frac{60 \text{ m\cancel{g}} \times 1 \text{ tsp}}{20 \text{ m\cancel{g}}} = \frac{20 \text{ \cancel{mg}} \times X}{20 \text{ \cancel{mg}}}$$

$$\frac{60 \text{ tsp}}{20} = X$$

$$3 \text{ tsp} = X$$

You should give the patient 3 tsp of phenobarbital elixir.

Quick quiz

1. One tablet of Lasix contains 40 mg, so three tablets contain:
   A.   120 mg.
   B.   150 mg.
   C.   180 mg.

Answer: A. If each tablet is 40 mg, multiply 40 by 3 to find the answer: 120 mg.

2. If a patient needs 100 mcg of Synthroid P.O. and the available dose is 25 mcg/tablet, the number of tablets to give is:
   A.   4.
   B.   6.
   C.   7.

Answer: A. If 1 tablet provides 25 mcg, divide 100 by 25 to get the answer: 4 tablets.

3. If 250 mg of Clozaril is ordered for a patient, but only 100-mg tablets are available, you should give:
   A.   2 tablets.
   B.   2½ tablets.
   C.   3½ tablets.

Answer: B. By dividing 250 by 100, you get 2.5, or 2½ tablets.

4. When reading a drug label, first check the:
   A.   dose strength.
   B.   generic name.
   C.   trade name.

Answer: B. The generic name follows the trade name on a drug label.

5. If the doctor orders *640 mg Tylenol liquid P.O. STAT* and the bottle label says Tylenol 80 mg per ½ tsp, you should give the patient:
   A.   15 ml.
   B.   20 ml.
   C.   25 ml.

Answer: B. First, consult a conversion table to find that 1 tsp equals 5 ml. Then use proportions to solve for X.

If you think these questions are hard now, back in the day, we didn't even have calculators!

6. If 80 mg of Lasix oral solution is ordered and Lasix 10 mg/ml is available, you should administer:

    A.   8 ml.

    B.   10 ml.

    C.   12 ml.

Answer: A. Use proportions to solve for *X*. Remember to use 1 ml as the known factor.

7. If a dose smaller than one-half of a scored tablet is needed, you should:

    A.   substitute a commercially available solution or suspension or one prepared by the pharmacist.

    B.   cut the tablet with a knife.

    C.   break the tablet with your hand.

Answer: A. Breaking an unscored tablet in portions smaller than one-half usually yields an incorrect dose.

8. Some drugs become unstable when they're supplied in powder form. Therefore, you must typically dilute them in which diluent before administration?

    A.   sterile water.

    B.   tap water.

    C.   normal saline solution.

Answer: B. Drugs that become unstable when they're stored as liquids are usually diluted with tap water before administration.

9. The doctor orders *30 mEq potassium chloride liquid q a.m. 3 days.* The only solution on hand contains 20 mEq 115 ml. How many milliliters should you give the patient?

    A.   23 ml

    B.   22 ml

    C.   20 ml

Answer: A. Use proportions to solve for *X*. Remember to round up to get your answer.

YES! Only one more question to go!

10. A patient needs 50 mg of Benadryl elixir P.O. STAT and the bottle label says Benadryl 12.5 mg/5 ml. You should give:

    A.   25 ml.
    B.   20 ml.
    C.   15 ml.

Answer: B. Use fractions to solve for *X*. The known factor is 12.5 mg equals 5 ml.

Scoring

★★★ If you answered all ten items correctly, excellent! Expressed as a ratio it's 9 : 9 :: 100 : 100 (in other words, perfect).

★★ If you answered seven to nine correctly, good job! Your calculation skills need practice (but, remember, a good calculator never hurt anybody).

★ If you answered fewer than seven correctly, don't worry! Keep on calculatin' (whether it's milligrams or milliliters).

Calculating topical and rectal drug dosages

Just the facts

In this chapter, you'll learn:

♦ how to interpret topical and rectal drug labels

♦ what types of drugs are given topically and rectally and how they work

♦ how to perform dosage calculations for topical and rectal drugs.

A look at topical and rectal drugs

Some types of drugs must be administered by the topical, or dermal, route. These drugs include creams, lotions, ointments, and powders, which commonly are used for dermatologic treatment or wound care, or patches, which have various uses, including treating angina. Topical drugs are applied to the skin and absorbed through the epidermis into the dermis.

Drugs also may be given rectally. This route may be best for patients who can't take drugs orally, such as those with nasogastric tubes, nausea, or vomiting. It also may be used for unconscious patients who can't swallow and to achieve specific local and systemic effects. Rectal drugs include enemas and suppositories.

Are you label able?

When you read the labels on topical and rectal drugs, look for the same information that you would with oral and parenteral drugs. (See *Labeling a successful administration*, page 164.)

The trade name appears first, followed by the generic name, the dose strength, and the total volume of the package. Labels also may contain special administration instructions. Sometimes, the

Before you give that drug!

Labeling a successful administration

There are three rules for administering medication: Read the label, read the label, read the label.

A topical topic

When reading a topical ointment label, note the following information as shown on the box label below:

- trade name (Bactroban)
- generic name (mupirocin)
- dose strength (2% ointment)
- total package volume (15 grams)
- special instructions (not included on this label).

Suppository story

When reading a rectal suppository label, note the following information as shown on the box label below:

- trade name (Compazine)
- generic name (prochlorperazine)
- dose strength (5 mg)
- total package volume (12 suppositories)
- special instructions (for older children [not under 40 lb]; for rectal use only).

print on the labels is quite small, so look carefully. (See *Combination product alert*.)

Transdermal patches

In the past, topical drugs were used almost solely for their local effects. Today, however, several topical drugs, such as transdermal patches, are used for their systemic effects as well.

I've got you under my skin

Transdermal patch drugs penetrate the outer layers of the skin by way of passive diffusion at a constant rate; then the drugs are absorbed into the circulation. Patches are a good way to administer drugs that aren't absorbed well in the GI tract as well as those that are metabolized and eliminated too quickly to be effective.

A patch dispatch

Patches are convenient and easy to use, and they maintain consistent blood levels of the drug. However, they also have disadvantages. Their onset of action is slow, so a therapeutic blood level takes hours or even days to achieve. Patches also need to be checked frequently, especially if the patient is active, because they may become displaced. In addition, reversing the toxic effects of patches can be difficult because the drug takes so long to be metabolized.

Release me

Drug concentrations in transdermal patches vary depending on the design of the patch, but the concentration isn't as important as the drug's rate of release. Two patches containing the same drug in different concentrations may actually release the same amount of drug per hour.

Batches of patches

Patches are available for a variety of conditions, including a nitroglycerin patch to prevent angina, a clonidine patch to control hypertension, and a fentanyl patch to manage chronic pain.

The fentanyl transdermal system, or Duragesic patch, is an example of a transdermal drug used systemically. It's held in a reservoir behind a membrane that allows controlled drug absorption through the skin. These patches are available in doses of 25, 50, 75, and 100 mcg/hour, with the higher doses for use with opioid-resistant patients. To ensure that the patient receives the correct dose, change the patch every 72 hours and check the label to verify the fentanyl dosage. (See *Prescribed patches*, page 166.)

Before you give that drug

Combination product alert

Topical preparations may contain more than one drug. For example, Mycitracin Plus ointment contains bacitracin, neomycin, polymyxin B, and lidocaine. Carefully note all ingredients when checking labels and make sure that your patient isn't allergic to any of them.

Patches are available for a variety of conditions.

Prescribed patches

The following transdermal drugs allow you to topically administer systemic drugs.

Nitroglycerin

Transdermal nitroglycerin provides prophylactic treatment of chronic angina. Available brands include Deponit, Nitrodisc, Nitro-Dur, and Transderm-Nitro. A new patch is applied daily (usually in the morning) and removed after 12 to 14 hours to prevent the patient from developing a tolerance to the drug.

Nicotine

Transdermal nicotine is used to treat smoking addiction. Brands include Habitrol, Nicoderm, Nicotrol, and ProStep. These drugs should be used only as adjuncts to behavioral therapy programs. A new patch is applied daily. Nicotrol should be removed after 16 hours, but other brands should stay on for 24 hours.

Fentanyl

Transdermal fentanyl is administered to treat severe chronic pain. Its brand name is Duragesic. Each patch may be worn as many as 72 hours.

Clonidine

Clonidine is used to treat hypertension. The brand name for this drug is Catapres TTS. A new patch is applied every 7 days.

Scopolamine

Scopolamine is used to treat nausea, vomiting, and vertigo. Brands include Transderm-Scōp and Transderm-V (available in Canada). The patch is applied to skin behind the ear at least 4 hours before an antiemetic effect is needed. It can be worn for 3 days.

Estradiol

Transdermal estradiol provides hormone replacement to estrogen-deficient women. The brand names include Climara, Estraderm, and Vivelle. It's administered on an intermittent cyclic schedule (3 weeks of therapy followed by discontinuation for 1 week).

Testosterone

Transdermal testosterone provides hormone replacement for men with testosterone deficiency. The brand names are Androderm and Testoderm. The Testoderm patch is applied once daily to clean, hairless scrotal skin, which is the only skin that's thin enough to allow adequate blood levels to be achieved.

Topical drug dosages

Determining topical drug dosages requires very little calculating. As previously discussed, transdermal patches are changed at regular intervals to ensure that the patient receives the correct dose. To apply a patch, simply remove the old patch and replace it with a new one at the appropriate time, following the manufacturer's guidelines.

Applying your judgment (along with the ointment)

When the doctor prescribes an ointment as part of wound care or dermatologic treatment, he usually leaves the amount to apply up to you. He may give general guidance, such as "use a thin layer" or

Cheat sheet

Topical drug calculations

• Use your own judgment in accordance with the doctor's general instructions.
• Follow specific guidelines for drugs prescribed for a systemic effect.

Peak technique

Measuring a topical dose

To measure a specified amount of ointment from a tube, squeeze the prescribed length of ointment in inches or centimeters onto a paper ruler like that shown here. Then use the ruler to apply the ointment to the patient's skin at the appropriate time, following the manufacturer's guidelines for administration.

Nitrol® Ointment
(Nitroglycerin Ointment USP, 2%)
APPLI-RULER®

INCHES   1/2   1   1 1/2   2

CENTIMETERS   1.25   2.5   3.75   5

the applicator that measures the dose

® Manufactured for:
SAVAGE LABORATORIES®
a division of Altana Inc.
MELVILLE, NEW YORK 11747
by: Altana Inc., MELVILLE, NEW YORK 11747

"apply thickly." When an ointment contains a drug intended for a systemic effect, more specific administration guidelines are necessary.

Many ointments, including nitroglycerin, are available in tubes. To apply ointment from a tube, use a paper ruler applicator to measure the correct dose. (See *Measuring a topical dose*.)

Rectal drug dosages

Rectal drugs include enemas and suppositories. Suppositories are the most common form of rectal drugs.

To calculate the number of suppositories to give, use the proportion method with ratios or fractions. The doctor usually prescribes drugs in the dose provided by one suppository, but occasionally you may need to insert two suppositories. (See *Check and check again*, page 168.)

the Real World

Real world problems

The problems below illustrate how to calculate suppository dosages.

Your pediatric patient needs 240 mg of acetaminophen by suppository. The package label reads *acetaminophen suppositories 120 mg*. How many suppositories should you give?

This is how to solve this problem using fractions.

• Set up the first fraction with the known suppository dose:

$$\frac{1 \text{ supp}}{120 \text{ mg}}$$

• Set up the second fraction with the desired dose and the unknown number of suppositories:

$$\frac{X}{240 \text{ mg}}$$

• Put these fractions into a proportion:

$$\frac{1 \text{ supp}}{120 \text{ mg}} = \frac{X}{240 \text{ mg}}$$

• Cross-multiply the fractions:

$$120 \text{ mg} \times X = 1 \text{ supp} \times 240 \text{ mg}$$

• Solve for X by dividing each side of the equation by 120 mg and canceling units that appear in both the numerator and denominator:

$$\frac{120 \cancel{\text{ mg}} \times X}{120 \cancel{\text{ mg}}} = \frac{1 \text{ supp} \times 240 \cancel{\text{ mg}}}{120 \cancel{\text{ mg}}}$$

$$X = 2 \text{ suppositories}$$

Suppose you calculate this suppository dose?

The doctor's order states *Dulcolax 10 mg per rectum at 6 a.m.* You only have 5-mg suppositories on hand. How many suppositories should you give this patient?

This is how to solve this using fractions.

• Set up the first fraction with the known suppository dose:

$$\frac{1 \text{ supp}}{5 \text{ mg}}$$

• Set up the second fraction with the desired dose and the unknown number of suppositories:

$$\frac{X}{10 \text{ mg}}$$

Check and check again

Occasionally you may need to insert more than one or a portion of one suppository. Here's what to do.

More than one

Do your dosage calculations indicate a need for more than one suppository? If so, check your figures and ask another nurse to check them, too. Then ask the pharmacist whether the suppository is available in other dosage strengths.

More than two

If more than two suppositories are needed, confirm the dose with the doctor. Then check with the pharmacist. He may be able to give you one suppository with an adequate amount of the drug.

A portion of one

If less than one suppository is needed, check your calculations and have another nurse do the same. Then ask the pharmacist if the dose is available in one suppository. This ensures the most accurate dose.

- Put these fractions into a proportion:

$$\frac{1 \text{ supp}}{5 \text{ mg}} = \frac{X}{10 \text{ mg}}$$

- Cross-multiply the fractions:

$$1 \text{ supp} \times 10 \text{ mg} = X \times 5 \text{ mg}$$

- Solve for X by dividing each side of the equation by 5 mg and canceling units that appear in both the numerator and denominator:

$$\frac{1 \text{ supp} \times 10 \text{ mg}}{5 \text{ mg}} = \frac{X \times 5 \text{ mg}}{5 \text{ mg}}$$

$$X = 2 \text{ suppositories}$$

Cheat sheet

Rectal drug calculations

- Use the proportion method with ratios or fractions.
- Dose is typically prescribed to be provided by one suppository (occasionally two).

A tiger of a Tigan problem

The doctor orders a 100-mg Tigan suppository for your patient. The pharmacy is closed, and the only Tigan on hand contains 200 mg per suppository. How many suppositories should you give?

This is how to solve this using ratios.

- Set up the first ratio with the known suppository dose:

$$1 \text{ supp} : 200 \text{ mg}$$

- Set up the second ratio with the desired dose and the unknown number of suppositories:

$$X : 100 \text{ mg}$$

- Put these ratios into a proportion:

$$1 \text{ supp} : 200 \text{ mg} :: X : 100 \text{ mg}$$

- Multiply the means and the extremes:

$$200 \text{ mg} \times X = 100 \text{ mg} \times 1 \text{ supp}$$

- Solve for X by dividing each side of the equation by 200 mg and canceling units that appear in both the numerator and denominator:

$$\frac{200 \text{ mg} \times X}{200 \text{ mg}} = \frac{100 \text{ mg} \times 1 \text{ supp}}{200 \text{ mg}}$$

$$X = \tfrac{1}{2} \text{ suppository}$$

Say it
100 times...
I love math...
I love math...
I love math...

Quick quiz

YIPPEEE! I'm finished (at least until the next chapter).

1. According to the label below, the generic name of this drug is:

    A.   Retin-A Gel.
    B.   tretinoin.
    C.   hydroxypropyl cellulose.

Answer: B. On drug labels, the generic name always appears in lowercase letters after the trade name.

2. Transdermal patches used to relieve chronic pain are effective for many hours due to:
    A.   controlled absorption through the skin.
    B.   enhanced effect on local tissue.
    C.   rapid then slow release of analgesics.

Answer: A. These drugs are slowly released and absorbed through the skin over a period of time.

3. A commonly used transdermal drug is:
    A.   Anectine.
    B.   nitroglycerin.
    C.   M S Contin.

Answer: B. Nitroglycerin patches are used to prevent angina.

4. If a drug label reads *Compazine (prochlorperazine) suppositories 5 mg, SmithKline Beecham, for rectal use only,* the drug's proprietary name is:
    A.   Compazine.
    B.   prochlorperazine.
    C.   SmithKline Beecham.

Answer: A. The proprietary name, or trade name, always appears first on a drug label.

5. If the doctor's order reads *Nitrol Ointment 1″ q6h*, you should measure this dose:
    A.   on a paper ruler applicator.
    B.   by using your own judgment to approximate 1″ of ointment.
    C.   by holding a wooden ruler to the patient's skin to measure the ointment.

Answer: A. Nitrol Ointment comes with its own paper ruler. Squeeze the prescribed length of ointment onto the ruler and then use the ruler to apply the ointment to the patient's skin.

6. If a patient needs 500 mg of aminophylline by suppository but all you have are 250-mg suppositories, you should insert:
    A.   1 suppository.
    B.   2 suppositories.
    C.   3 suppositories.

Answer: B. A simple calculation tells you that the patient needs 2 suppositories. However, because more than 1 suppository is needed, you should check your calculations, have another nurse do the same, and then call the pharmacy to see if a 500-mg dose is available.

7. When a doctor prescribes an antibiotic ointment for a finger laceration, you should:
    A.   ask him to prescribe a specific amount.
    B.   use a paper applicator to apply the ointment.
    C.   use your own judgment about the amount of ointment to apply.

Answer: C. Unless the ointment has a systemic effect, the doctor will usually leave the amount to apply up to you.

8. If a child needs 2.5 mg of Compazine, and the package label reads *Compazine suppositories 5 mg*, you should give:
    A.   2 suppositories.
    B.   ½ suppository.
    C.   1 suppository.

Answer: B. By setting up a proportion and solving for *X*, you'll find that the child needs ½ of a 5-mg suppository.

9. Your patient is receiving transdermal nitroglycerin for treatment of angina. Which action is necessary when administering this drug?

    A.   Remove the patch after 7 days.

    B.   Remove the patch after 72 hours.

    C.   Remove the patch after 12 to 14 hours.

Answer: C. Transdermal nitroglycerin should be removed after 12 to 14 hours to prevent the patient from developing a tolerance to the drug.

Scoring

☆☆☆ If you answered all nine items correctly, wow! You know your routes better than AAA!

☆☆ If you answered six to eight correctly, all right! You'll soon be top dog in topical drug administration!

☆ If you answered fewer than six correctly, keep at it! You're absorbing information at an incredible rate!

Part V

Parenteral administration

11 Calculating parenteral injections 175

12 Calculating I.V. infusions 205

Calculating parenteral injections

Just the facts

In this chapter, you'll learn:

♦ about calculating intradermal, subcutaneous, and intra-muscular injections

♦ about different types of syringes and needles

♦ how to interpret parenteral drug labels

♦ how to administer insulin therapy

♦ how to reconstitute powders.

A look at parenteral injections

Parenteral is a term that refers to "outside the intestines." Drugs may be administered parenterally through direct injection into the skin, subcutaneous tissue, muscle, or vein. They may be supplied as liquids or as powders that require reconstitution. When using either form, you need to perform calculations to determine the amount of liquid medication to inject.

This chapter shows how to use the ratio and proportion method to calculate liquid parenteral dosages, as well as how to reconstitute powdered drugs. Another parenteral drug administration route, I.V. infusion, is discussed in the next chapter. I.V. injections are discussed in chapter 15, Calculating critical care dosages.

Types of injections

Parenteral drugs are administered by four types of injections:
• intradermal
• subcutaneous (S.C.)

- intramuscular (I.M.)
- I.V. (See chapter 12, Calculating I.V. infusions.).

Giving parenteral drugs safely depends on choosing the right type of injection for the patient's condition and the right syringe and needle for the type of injection.

Intradermal injections

In an intradermal injection, medication is injected into the dermis—the layer of skin beneath the epidermis, or the outermost layer of skin. This type of injection is used to anesthetize the skin for invasive procedures and to test for allergies, tuberculosis, histoplasmosis, and other diseases.

I've got you intra my skin.

The volume of a drug that's given by intradermal injection is less than 0.5 ml. A 1-ml syringe, calibrated in 0.01-ml increments, is usually used, along with a 25- to 27-gauge (G) needle that's ⅜″ to ⅝″ long.

To perform an intradermal injection, use this basic procedure:

☝   Clean the skin thoroughly.

✌   Stretch the skin taut with one hand.

🤟   With your other hand, insert the needle quickly at a 10- to 15-degree angle to a depth of about 0.5 cm.

🖐   Inject the drug. A small wheal forms where the drug is injected into the skin.

Subcutaneous injections

In an S.C. injection, the drug is injected into the subcutaneous tissue, which is beneath the dermis and above the muscle. Drugs are absorbed faster in this layer than in the dermis because this layer has more capillaries. Insulin, heparin, tetanus toxoid, and some narcotics are injected through this route.

More than skin deep

Only 0.5 to 1.5 ml of a drug can be injected S.C. The needles used for S.C. injections are 23G to 28G and ½″ to ⅝″ long. S.C. injection sites include the:
- lateral areas of the upper arms and thighs
- abdomen (above, below, and lateral to the umbilicus)
- upper back.

Make sure the patient's skin is good and clean!

To perform an S.C. injection, use this basic procedure:
- Choose the injection site.
- Clean the skin.
- If the patient is thin, pinch the skin between your index finger and thumb, and insert the needle at a 45-degree angle.
- If the patient is obese, insert the needle into the fatty tissue at a 90-degree angle.
- Aspirate for blood (unless injecting insulin or heparin).
- Administer the injection.
- Massage the site after removing the needle; this may enhance absorption. Don't massage site if you're giving heparin or insulin.

Intramuscular injections

An I.M. injection, which goes into a muscle, is used for drugs that need to be absorbed quickly, that are given in a large volume, or that irritate the tissues if given by a shallow route. The volume for these injections ranges from 0.5 to 3 ml. I.M. injection sites include the:
- ventral gluteal or vastus lateralis muscle (for 3-ml injections)
- rectus femoris or deltoid muscle (for injections of less than 3 ml).

The choice of injection site depends on the patient's muscle mass and overlying tissue and the volume of the injection. The needles are 1″ to 3″ long, and are 18G to 23G in diameter.

Use a little muscle.

To administer an I.M. injection, use this basic procedure:
- Choose the injection site.
- Clean the skin.
- Using a quick, dartlike action, insert the needle at a 75- to 90-degree angle.
- Before injecting the drug, aspirate for blood to make sure the needle isn't in a vein.
- Push the plunger and keep the syringe steady.
- After the drug is injected, pull the needle straight out and apply pressure to the site.

Syringes and needles

The several types of syringes and needles used to administer parenteral drugs are designed for specific purposes.

Cheat sheet

S.C. injections

- Common drugs — insulin, heparin, tetanus toxoid, some narcotics
- Drug's volume — 0.5 to 1.5 ml
- Needle — 23G to 28G, ½″ to ⅝″ in length

Insulin and heparin S.C. injections
- Don't aspirate for blood
- Don't massage site

Cheat sheet

I.M. injections

- Drugs needing quick absorption or those that are irritating to tissue
- Drugs's volume 0.5 to 3 ml
- Needles — 18G to 23G, 1″ to 3″ in length

Before injection
- Aspirate for blood to make sure needle isn't in vein

Types of syringes

To measure and administer parenteral drugs, three basic types of hypodermic syringes are used:
- standard syringes
- tuberculin syringes
- prefilled syringes.

Although these syringes are sometimes calibrated in cubic centimeters, the drugs they're used to measure are commonly ordered in milliliters. (Recall that 1 cc equals 1 ml and that milliliters and cubic centimeters are used interchangeably.)

Standard syringes

Standard syringes are available in 3, 5, 10, 20, 30, 50, and 60 ml. Each syringe consists of a plunger, a barrel, a hub, a needle, and dead space. The dead space holds fluid that remains in the syringe and needle after the plunger is completely depressed. Some syringes, such as insulin syringes, don't have dead space. (See *Anatomy of a syringe.*)

Marked for good measure

The calibration marks on syringes allow you to accurately measure drug doses. The 3-ml syringe, the most commonly used, is calibrated in tenths of a milliliter on the right and minims on the

Anatomy of a syringe

Standard syringes come in many different sizes, but each syringe has the same components. This illustration shows the parts of a standard syringe.

left. It has large marks for 0.5 ml on the right. The large-volume syringes are calibrated in 2- to 10-ml increments.

To administer a drug, remember the "five rights" of medication administration — right drug, right route, right dose, right time, right patient — then follow these basic steps:

- Use aseptic technique.
- Calculate the dose.
- Draw the drug into the syringe.
- Pull the plunger back until the top ring of the plunger's black portion aligns with the correct calibration mark.
- Double-check the dose measurement.
- Administer the drug.

Double the fun (well, not exactly fun)

Parenteral drugs come in various dose strengths or concentrations so that the usual adult dose can be contained in 1 to 3 ml of solution. If a patient needs a dose larger than 3 ml, give it in two injections at two different sites to ensure proper drug absorption.

Tuberculin syringes

Tuberculin syringes are commonly used for intradermal injections and to administer small amounts of drugs, such those given as to pediatric patients or those on intensive care units. Each syringe is calibrated in hundredths of a milliliter on the right and minims on the left, allowing you to accurately administer doses as small as 0.25 ml. Tuberculin syringes are also marked for alternate tenths of a milliliter: 0.2, 0.4, 0.6, and 0.8 ml. (See *Touring a tuberculin syringe*, page 180.)

Read the fine print

Measure drugs in a tuberculin syringe as you would those in with a standard syringe. Take extra care when reading the dose, however, because the measurements on the tuberculin syringe are very small.

Prefilled syringes

A sterile syringe filled with a premeasured dose of drug is called a prefilled syringe. These syringes usually come with a cartridge-needle unit and require a special holder called a Carpuject or Tubex to release the drug from the cartridge. Each cartridge is calibrated in tenths of a milliliter and has larger marks for half and full milliliters. (See *Presenting a prefilled syringe*, page 181.)

If a patient needs a dose larger than 3 ml, give it in two injections at different sites to ensure absorption.

Room for one more

Some cartridges are designed so that a diluent or a second drug can be added when a combined dose is ordered. For example, many narcotics, such as meperidine (Demerol), come from the manufacturer in prefilled syringes. Because Demerol is often ordered along with hydroxyzine (Vistaril), the Demerol cartridge allows for the addition of Vistaril. *Always check a compatibility chart when mixing more than one drug in a syringe.*

First, the good news...

Prefilled syringes have many advantages over multiple-dose vials. Because they're labeled with the drug name and dose, preparation time is reduced and so is the risk of drug errors.

This labeling also makes it easier to record the amount of drug used and eliminates the need to figure out how much drug is left in a vial after you've given an injection. This is especially important with narcotic doses, which the law says must be recorded exactly.

The most obvious advantage of prefilled syringes is that you don't have to measure each drug dose. The manufacturer has already done this and placed the dose in the syringe. *However, be aware that most manufacturers add a little extra drug to the syringe in case some is wasted when the syringe is purged of air.*

Touring a tuberculin syringe

A tuberculin syringe has the same components as a standard syringe. However, size and calibration of the syringe are distinct. Because the measurements on the tuberculin syringe are so small, take extra care when reading the dose.

Dead space
Barrel
Needle
Hub
Plunger

...Now, the bad news

Unfortunately, prefilled syringes aren't available in all doses. When the ordered dose doesn't match the amount in the prefilled syringe, you'll need to calculate the correct amount of drug needed.

After giving the injection, discard the extra drug by expelling it from the syringe. If the drug is a narcotic, document carefully the amount of drug you discard. Have another nurse witness the expulsion of the drug and then co-sign the narcotic record.

Closed-system devices

Another type of prefilled syringe, a closed-system device, comes with a needle and syringe in place and a separate prefilled drug chamber. Emergency drugs, such as atropine and lidocaine, come in this type of prefilled syringe.

To prepare a closed-system device, hold the drug chamber in one hand and the syringe and needle in the other. Flip the protective caps off both ends. Insert the drug chamber into the syringe section. Then remove the needle cap and expel air and extra medication.

Presenting a prefilled syringe

This illustration shows the parts of a prefilled syringe. Take note of the holder at right. The most commonly used brands of prefilled syringes are Carpuject and Tubex.

Types of needles

Five types of needles are used to inject drugs: intradermal, subcutaneous, intramuscular, intravenous, and filter. Each type of needle is designed for a different purpose. (See *Choosing the right needle.*)

When choosing a needle, consider the gauge, bevel, and length:
• Gauge refers to the inside diameter of the needle; the smaller the gauge, the larger the diameter. For example, a 14G needle has a larger diameter than a 25G needle.
• Bevel refers to the angle at which the needle tip is opened. The bevel may be short, medium, or long.
• Length describes the distance from needle tip to needle hub. It ranges from $^3/_8''$ to 3".

Choosing the right needle

When choosing a needle, consider its purpose as well as its gauge, bevel, and length. Use the following selection guide to choose the right needles for your patients.

Intradermal needles
Intradermal needles are $^3/_8''$ to $^5/_8''$ long, usually have short bevels, and are 25G to 27G in diameter.

Subcutaneous needles
Subcutaneous needles are $^1/_2''$ to $^5/_8''$ long, have medium bevels, and are 23G to 28G in diameter.

Intramuscular needles
Intramuscular needles are 1" to 3" long, have medium bevels, and are 18G to 23G in diameter.

Intravenous needle
Intravenous needles are 1" to 3" long, have long bevels, and are 14G to 25G in diameter.

Filter needles
Filter needles are used for preparing a solution from a vial or ampule and shouldn't be used for injections. They're $1^1/_2''$ long, have medium bevels, and are 20G in diameter.

Microscopic pieces of rubber or glass can enter the solution when you puncture the diaphragm of a vial with a needle or snap open an ampule. You can use a filter needle with a screening device in the hub to remove minute particles of foreign material from a solution. After the medication is prepared, discard the filter needle.

Real world problems

The following examples show how to use the proportion method to calculate doses given by injection.

Prefilled painkiller problem

The doctor prescribes *4 mg of I.M. morphine every 3 hours* for your patient's pain. The drug is available in a prefilled syringe containing 10 mg of morphine/ml. How many milliliters of morphine should you waste?

This is how to solve this problem using fractions:

• Set up the first fraction using the known morphine dose:

$$\frac{10 \text{ mg}}{1 \text{ ml}}$$

• Set up the second fraction with the desired dose and the unknown amount of morphine:

$$\frac{4 \text{ mg}}{X}$$

• Put these fractions into a proportion:

$$\frac{10 \text{ mg}}{1 \text{ ml}} = \frac{4 \text{ mg}}{X}$$

• Cross-multiply the fractions:

$$10 \text{ mg} \times X = 4 \text{ mg} \times 1 \text{ ml}$$

• Solve for X by dividing each side of the equation by 10 mg and canceling units that appear in both the numerator and denominator:

$$\frac{\cancel{10 \text{ mg}} \times X}{\cancel{10 \text{ mg}}} = \frac{4 \cancel{\text{ mg}} \times 1 \text{ ml}}{10 \cancel{\text{ mg}}}$$

$$X = \frac{4 \text{ ml}}{10}$$

$$X = 0.4 \text{ ml}$$

• The amount of morphine to give the patient is 0.4 ml. To calculate the amount to be wasted, subtract the ordered dose from the entire contents of the syringe:

$$
\begin{array}{rl}
1.0 \text{ ml} = & 10 \text{ mg morphine} \\
- \ 0.4 \text{ ml} = & 4 \text{ mg morphine} \\
\hline
0.6 \text{ ml} = & 6 \text{ mg morphine}
\end{array}
$$

The amount of morphine to be wasted is 0.6 ml.

Medrol milligram mystery

The doctor orders *100 mg of methylprednisolone (Solu-Medrol) I.M. every 4 hours* for your patient with asthma. The vial contains 120 mg/ml. How much Solu-Medrol should you give?

This is how to solve this problem using ratios:
- Set up the first ratio with the known Solu-Medrol dose:

$$120 \text{ mg} : 1 \text{ ml}$$

- Set up the second ratio with the desired dose and the unknown amount of Solu-Medrol:

$$100 \text{ mg} : X$$

- Put these ratios into a proportion:

$$120 \text{ mg} : 1 \text{ ml} :: 100 \text{ mg} : X$$

- Set up an equation by multiplying the extremes and the means:

$$120 \text{ mg} \times X = 100 \text{ mg} \times 1 \text{ ml}$$

- Solve for X by dividing each side of the equation by 120 mg and canceling units that appear in both the numerator and denominator:

$$\frac{120 \text{ mg} \times X}{120 \text{ mg}} = \frac{100 \text{ mg} \times 1 \text{ ml}}{120 \text{ mg}}$$

$$X = \frac{100 \text{ ml}}{120}$$

$$X = 0.83 \text{ ml}$$

You should give the patient 0.83 ml of Solu-Medrol.

Vial trial

The doctor prescribes *100 mg of gentamicin I.M.* for your patient. The vial available contains 40 mg/ml. How much gentamicin should you give?

This is how to solve this problem using ratios:
- Set up the first ratio with the known gentamicin dose:

$$40 \text{ mg} : 1 \text{ ml}$$

- Set up the second ratio with the desired dose and the unknown amount of gentamicin:

$$100 \text{ mg} : X$$

- Put these ratios into a proportion:

$$40 \text{ mg} : 1 \text{ ml} :: 100 \text{ mg} : X$$

- Set up an equation by multiplying the means and the extremes:

$$1 \text{ ml} \times 100 \text{ mg} = 40 \text{ mg} \times X$$

- Solve for X by dividing each side of the equation by 40 mg and canceling units that appear in both the numerator and denominator:

$$\frac{1 \text{ ml} \times 100 \text{ mg}}{40 \text{ mg}} = \frac{40 \text{ mg} \times X}{40 \text{ mg}}$$

$$\frac{100 \text{ ml}}{40} = X$$

$$X = 2.5 \text{ ml}$$

You should give the patient 2.5 ml of gentamicin.

Interpreting drug labels

Before you can safely administer a parenteral drug, you must know how to read its label. (See *A close look at labels*.) Parenteral drugs are packaged in glass ampules, in single- or multiple-dose

A close look at labels

The labels below show all the information you need to safely administer a parenteral drug.

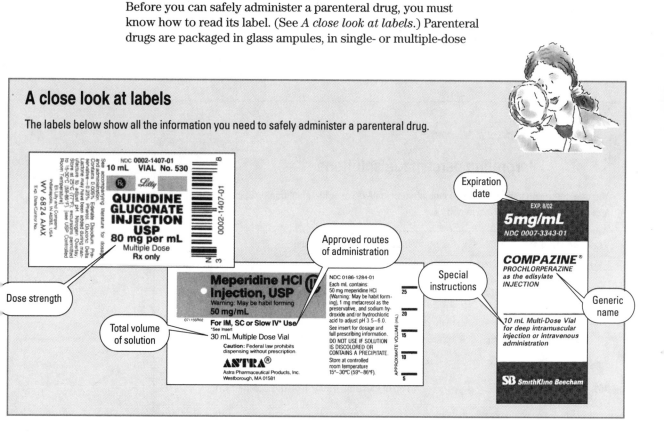

vials with rubber stoppers, and in prefilled syringes and cartridges.

Looking at labels

Reading the label of a parenteral solution is a lot like reading an oral solution label. This is the information you'll see:
- trade name
- generic name
- total volume of solution in the container
- dose strength or concentration (drug dose present in a volume of solution)
- expiration date
- special instructions, as needed.

Cheat sheet

Solute or solution?

- Solute — a drug in liquid or solid form
- Solution — liquid (usually sterile water) with a dissolved solute

Percentage and ratio solutions

A solute is a liquid or solid form of a drug. A solution is a liquid that contains a solute dissolved in a diluent or solvent, most often sterile water. Normal saline solution is a solution of salt (the solute) in purified water (the solvent). Solutions come in different strengths, which are expressed on the drug label as percentage solutions or ratio solutions.

What does it all mean?

Interpreting percentage solutions

You can determine the contents of a weight/volume (W/V) or volume/volume (V/V) percentage solution by reading the label, as shown here.

What the label says	What the solution contains
0.9% (W/V) NaCl	0.9 g of sodium chloride in 100 ml of finished solution
5% (W/V) boric acid solution	5 g of boric acid in 100 ml of finished solution
5% (W/V) dextrose	5 g of dextrose in 100 ml of finished solution
2% (V/V) hydrogen peroxide	2 ml of hydrogen peroxide in 100 ml of finished solution
70% (V/V) isopropyl alcohol	70 ml of isopropyl alcohol in 100 ml of finished solution
10% (V/V) glycerin	10 ml of glycerin in 100 ml of finished solution

What does it all mean?

Interpreting ratio solutions

You can determine the contents of a weight per volume (W : V) or volume per volume (V : V) ratio solution from the label, as shown here.

What the label says	What the solution contains
benzalkonium chloride 1 : 750 (W : V)	1 g of benzalkonium chloride in 750 ml of finished solution
silver nitrate 1 : 100 (W : V)	1 g of silver nitrate in 100 ml of finished solution
hydrogen peroxide 2 : 100 (V : V)	2 ml of hydrogen peroxide in 100 ml of finished solution
glycerin 10 : 100 (V : V)	10 ml of glycerin in 100 ml of finished solution

Perusing percentages

A clear way to label or describe a solution is as a percentage. Providing information in percentages makes it easy to make dosage calculations, dilutions, or alterations. (See *Interpreting percentage solutions.*)

Interpreting solutions

On the label, a solution may be expressed either as weight per volume (W/V) or volume per volume (V/V).

In a weight per volume solution, the percentage or strength refers to the number of grams (the weight) of solute per 100 ml (the volume) of finished, or reconstituted, solution. With volume per volume, the percentage refers to the number of milliliters of solute per 100 ml of finished solution.

Here's how to express these two relationships mathematically:

$$\% = \frac{\text{weight}}{\text{volume}} = \text{grams solute/100 ml finished solution}$$

$$\% = \frac{\text{volume}}{\text{volume}} = \text{milliliters solute/100 ml finished solution}$$

Reviewing ratios

Another way to label or describe a solution is as a ratio. (See *Interpreting ratio solutions.*) The strength of a ratio solution usually is expressed as two numbers separated by a colon. In a weight

Cheat sheet

Ratio solutions

• W : V solutions: First number is the amount of the drug in grams. The second number is the volume of finished solution in milliliters.
• V : V solutions: First number is the amount of the drug in millimeters. The second number is the volume of finished solution in millimeters.

per volume solution (W:V), the first number signifies the amount of a drug in grams. In a volume per volume (V:V) solution, the first number signifies the amount of drug in milliliters. The second number signifies the volume of finished solution in milliliters.

This relationship is expressed as:

Ratio = amount of drug : amount of finished solution

Insulin and insulin therapy

Some drugs, such as insulin, heparin, and penicillin G, are measured in units. The unit system is based on an international standard of drug potency, not on weight. The number of units appears on the drug label. (See *Look for the unit label.*)

Insulin, a potent hormone produced by the pancreas, regulates carbohydrate metabolism. The effect of insulin's activity is reflected in blood glucose levels. A lack of insulin causes diabetes.

Insulin injections

Insulin is injected S.C. in patients with chronic diabetes or I.V. in patients with acute diabetic ketoacidosis. You must calculate and administer insulin doses carefully because even a small error can cause a hypoglycemic or hyperglycemic reaction.

Types of diabetes

There are two major types of diabetes: type 1 and type 2. Type 1 diabetes typically is diagnosed in patients younger than age 20 and requires long-term insulin therapy.

Type 2 diabetes usually is diagnosed in patients older than age 40; however, its incidence among children is rising. Type 2 diabetes can be controlled by diet and oral antidiabetic agents, although insulin may be used occasionally to stabilize blood glucose levels.

Types of insulin

Several types of insulin are available. The doctor chooses a particular type based on the patient's diet and activity level and the severity of disease.

Insulin origins

Insulin is classified according to its origin (human or animal) and action time. Some insulins are derived from pork pancreas and

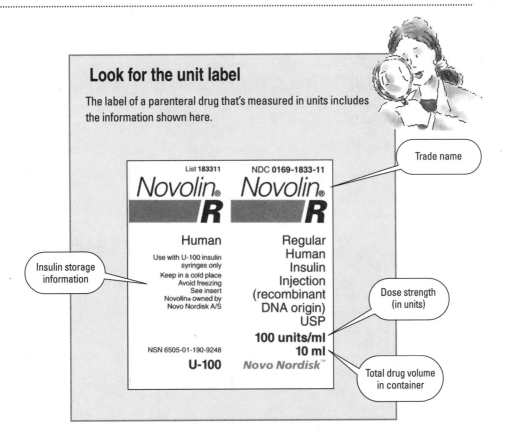

Look for the unit label

The label of a parenteral drug that's measured in units includes the information shown here.

Trade name

Insulin storage information

List **183311**

NDC **0169-1833-11**

Novolin® *Novolin*®

R **R**

Human

Use with U-100 insulin syringes only
Keep in a cold place
Avoid freezing
See insert
Novolin® owned by
Novo Nordisk A/S

NSN 6505-01-190-9248

U-100

Regular
Human
Insulin
Injection
(recombinant
DNA origin)
USP

100 units/ml
10 ml

Novo Nordisk™

Dose strength (in units)

Total drug volume in container

differ from human insulin by only two amino acids. Others are identical to human insulin and are produced by enzymatic conversion of pork insulin or by recombinant deoxyribonucleic acid techniques. The origin appears on the drug label.

Insulin initials

Most insulin labels also contain an initial after the trade name, indicating the type of insulin. These different types of insulin vary with regard to onset, peak, and duration of action. The initials are:
• R for regular insulin
• L for lente insulin
• U for ultralente insulin
• N for neutral protamine Hagedorn (NPH) insulin. (See *Reading insulin labels*, page 190, and *Identifying insulin subtypes*, page 191.)

Each in its own time

Insulin preparations are modified by combination with larger, insoluble protein molecules to slow absorption and prolong activity. Thus, the different types of insulin vary with regard to pharmacokinetic properties. (See *Insulin action times*, page 192.)

Remember to read insulin labels carefully.

Before you give that drug!

Reading insulin labels

Read insulin labels carefully to find the information you need for safe administration. Note that the origin or source of insulin is printed on every label.

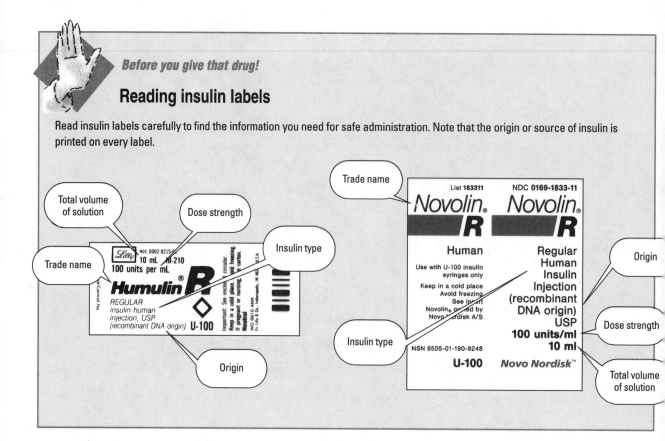

What dose do U want?

Insulin doses, expressed in units (U), are available in two concentrations. U-100 insulin, which contains 100 U of insulin per milliliter, is called universal because it's the most common concentration. U-500 insulin, which contains 500 U/ml, is used on rare occasions when a patient needs an unusually large dose.

Insulin syringes

A U-100 syringe, the only type of insulin syringe available in the United States, is calibrated so that 1 ml holds 100 U of insulin. A low-dose U-100 syringe, holding 50 U of insulin or less, is also used for some patients.

Because no syringes are made for it, U-500 insulin must also be administered with a U-100 syringe. Therefore, exercise caution when administering this drug. (See *Selecting an insulin syringe*, page 193.)

Reading insulin orders

Some patients' insulin doses are based on home monitoring of blood glucose values with glucometers. When a diagnosis of diabetes is first made, however, the patient undergoes tests to determine blood and urine glucose levels. Usually, the patient is enrolled in an outpatient center where he can be educated about diet, exercise, monitoring of blood glucose levels, and administration of insulin. Blood and urine glucose baselines are established.

Based on these determinations, the doctor may order small doses of rapid-acting insulin to be given at set times, such as every 4 hours or before meals and at bedtime, for several days. After a stable 24-hour dosage has been determined, the doctor may order dosage adjustments, such as one or two daily doses of intermediate-

Cheat sheet

Insulin doses

- Measured in units
- Based on drug potency (not weight)
- Classified as to origin and action time
- Universal concentration — U-100 insulin

Before you give that drug!

Identifying insulin subtypes

Insulin labels must be read carefully because they may contain confusingly similar information. Remember that one type of insulin, such as lente, may come in different subtypes but that those subtypes aren't interchangeable. For example, if the doctor prescribes lente human insulin zinc suspension, don't substitute lente purified pork insulin zinc suspension USP. Otherwise a hypersensitive patient could develop a severe allergic reaction.

Type	Subtype
Lente	• Lente human insulin zinc suspension (semisynthetic) • Lente purified pork insulin zinc suspension USP
NPH	• NPH human insulin isophane suspension USP • NPH purified pork isophane insulin suspension USP • 70% NPH, human insulin isophane suspension and 30% regular, human insulin injection (semisynthetic)
Regular	• Regular human insulin injection (semisynthetic) USP • Regular insulin, insulin injection USP (pork) • Regular purified pork insulin injection USP
Ultralente	• Ultralente insulin, extended insulin zinc suspension USP • Ultralente human extended zinc insulin suspension

Wow! That's a lot of subtypes.

Insulin action times

Insulin preparations are modified through combination with larger insoluble protein molecules to slow absorption and prolong activity. An insulin preparation may be rapid acting, intermediate acting, or long acting, as shown in the table below.

Drug	Onset	Peak	Duration
Rapid acting			
regular insulin	½ hr	2 to 4 hr	6 to 8 hr
lispro insulin	< ½ hr	½ to 1½ hr	< 6 hr
Intermediate acting			
insulin zinc suspension (lente)	1 to 3 hr	6 to 15 h	18 to 24 hr
isophane insulin suspension (NPH)	1 to 2 hr	4 to 12 hr	18 to 24 hr
isophane 70%, regular insulin 30%	½ hr	2 to 12 hr	24 hr
isophane 50%, regular insulin 50%	½ hr	4 to 8 hr	24 hr
Long acting			
extended insulin zinc suspension (ultralente)	4 to 6 hr	10 to 30 hr	24 to 36 hr
protamine zinc insulin suspension (PZI)			36 hr

acting insulin, possibly accompanied by small doses of rapid-acting insulin.

Insulin on a sliding scale

For a newly diagnosed, ill, or unstable diabetic patient, the doctor may write an order on a sliding scale. This type of order individualizes the insulin doses and administration times according to the patient's age, activity level, work habits, desired degree of blood glucose level control, and response to insulin preparations.

Selecting an insulin syringe

These two syringes are examples of the different dose-specific insulin syringes that are available. The U-100 syringe delivers up to 100 U of insulin. The low-dose syringe delivers up to 50 U of U-100 insulin.

U-100

Low-dose

This is an example of such an order:

Start regular insulin sliding scale:

Blood glucose values:	Insulin dose:
< 180 mg/dl	No insulin
180 to 240 mg/dl	10 U regular insulin S.C.
241 to 400 mg/dl	20 U regular insulin S.C.
> 400 mg/dl	Call doctor for orders.

Making connections with the dots

When reading insulin orders, check closely for decimal points that indicate unusual doses. (See *Danger! Disappearing decimal points,* page 194.)

If an order doesn't include the dose strength, then administer U-100 insulin, the universal strength. If U-500 insulin is needed, the doctor specifies this on the order.

Combining insulins

Sometimes the doctor will order regular insulin mixed with NPH insulin to be injected together at the same site. When you receive an order for these drugs, draw them into the same syringe, following this procedure:

Memory jogger

If you have trouble remembering which insulin to draw first, think of the phrase "clear before cloudy." (Who doesn't prefer a clear day to a cloudy day?)

This phrase also reminds you how these drugs work: A clear day seems short, but a cloudy day seems to go on forever. Clear, regular insulin is short-acting and cloudy. NPH insulin is long-acting.

- Read the insulin order carefully.
- Read the vial labels carefully, noting the type, concentration, source, and expiration date of the drugs.
- Roll the NPH vial between your palms to mix it thoroughly.
- Choose the appropriate syringe.
- Clean the tops of both vials of insulin with alcohol swabs.
- Inject air into the NPH vial equal to the amount of insulin you need to give. Withdraw the needle and syringe, but don't withdraw any NPH insulin.
- Inject into the regular insulin vial an amount of air equal to the dose of the regular insulin. Then invert or tilt the vial and withdraw the prescribed amount of regular insulin into the syringe. Draw the clear, regular insulin first to avoid contamination by the cloudy, longer-acting insulin.
- Clean the top of the NPH vial again. Then insert the needle of the syringe containing the regular insulin into the vial, and withdraw the prescribed amount of NPH insulin.
- Mix the insulins in the syringe by pulling back slightly on the plunger and tilting the syringe back and forth.
- Recheck the drug order, and administer the insulin immediately.

Real world problems

Before drawing up and administering insulin, heparin, or other drugs measured in units, check all your calculations for accuracy. The section that follows shows how to use the proportion method and a sliding scale to calculate insulin and heparin doses. (See *Heparin hazards*.)

Help! How much heparin?

The doctor orders *7,000 U of heparin S.C. q 12 h.* The heparin you have available contains 10,000 U/ml. How many milliliters of heparin should you give?

This is the calculation using ratios:

- Set up the first ratio with the known heparin dose:

$$10,000 \text{ U} : 1 \text{ ml}$$

- Set up the second ratio with the desired dose and the unknown amount of heparin:

$$7,000 \text{ U} : X$$

- Put these ratios into a proportion:

$$10,000 \text{ U} : 1 \text{ ml} :: 7,000 \text{ U} : X$$

Before you give that drug

Danger! Disappearing decimal points

When reading insulin orders, be alert to the placement of decimal points. Some patients are extremely sensitive to insulin, requiring a dose less than 10 U. To clarify this, the doctor may write the dose with a decimal point.

For example, the doctor may prescribe 3 U of insulin and write it as 3.0 U for clarity. If the decimal point is mistakenly lost during your transcription, the patient could receive 30 U of insulin, a tenfold dosing error. *If a dose seems unusually large or small, double-check it.*

- Set up an equation by multiplying the means and the extremes:

$$1 \text{ ml} \times 7,000 \text{ U} = 10,000 \text{ U} \times X$$

- Solve for X by dividing each side of the equation by 10,000 U and canceling units that appear in both the numerator and denominator:

$$\frac{1 \text{ ml} \times 7,000 \cancel{U}}{10,000 \cancel{U}} = \frac{\cancel{10,000 \text{ U}} \times X}{\cancel{10,000 \text{ U}}}$$

$$X = 0.7 \text{ ml}$$

You should give the patient 0.7 ml of heparin.

U-nsure about insulin?

The doctor prescribes *20 U of U-100 regular insulin.* The only syringe on hand is a 1-ml tuberculin syringe. How many milliliters should you administer?

This is the calculation using fractions:

- Set up the first fraction with the known insulin dose:

$$\frac{20 \text{ U}}{100 \text{ U}}$$

- Set up the second fraction with the unknown amount of insulin in milliliters and the desired dose:

$$\frac{X}{1 \text{ ml}}$$

- Put these fractions into a proportion:

$$\frac{20 \text{ U}}{100 \text{ U}} = \frac{X}{1 \text{ ml}}$$

- Cross-multiply the fractions:

$$100 \text{ U} \times X = 20 \text{ U} \times 1 \text{ ml}$$

- Solve for X by dividing each side of the equation by 100 U and canceling units that appear in both the numerator and denominator:

$$\frac{\cancel{100 \text{ U}} \times X}{\cancel{100 \text{ U}}} = \frac{20 \cancel{U} \times 1 \text{ ml}}{100 \cancel{U}}$$

$$X = 0.2 \text{ ml}$$

You should give the patient 0.2 ml of regular insulin.

Before you give that drug

Heparin hazards

The anticoagulant heparin is used in moderate doses to prevent thrombosis and embolism, and in large doses to treat these disorders. Heparin comes in many concentrations. Make sure that the heparin concentration is appropriate for the intended use.

Dosage calculation errors with heparin can cause excessive bleeding or undertreatment of a clotting disorder.

Another dosage calculation under my belt!

Insulin sliding scale

Insulin doses may be based on blood glucose levels, as shown in this table.

Blood glucose level	Insulin dose
< 200 mg/dl	No insulin
201 to 250 mg/dl	2 U regular insulin
251 to 300 mg/dl	4 U regular insulin
301 to 350 mg/dl	6 U regular insulin
351 to 400 mg/dl	8 U regular insulin
> 400 mg/dl	Call doctor for insulin order.

Insulin on a sliding scale

Your patient's blood glucose is 384 mg/dl. Based on the sliding scale below, how much insulin should you give him? (See *Insulin sliding scale*.)

You should administer 8 U of regular insulin.

Reconstituting powders

Some drugs— such as levothyroxine sodium (Synthroid) and penicillins— are manufactured and packaged as powders because they become unstable quickly when they're in solution. When the doctor prescribes such a drug, either you or the pharmacist must reconstitute it before it can be administered.

The strength of one or many

Powders come in single-strength or multiple-strength formulations. A single-strength powder— such as levothyroxine sodium— may be reconstituted to only one dose strength per administration route, as specified by the manufacturer. A multiple-strength powder— such as penicillins— can be reconstituted to various dose strengths by adjusting the amounts of diluent.

When reconstituting a multiple-strength powder, check the drug label or package insert for the dose-strength options and choose the one that's closest to the ordered dose strength.

Cheat sheet

Powders

• The fluid volume increases with the added diluent.

Single-strength
• Reconstitute these powders to one dose strength per administration route.

Multiple-strength
• Reconstitute these powders to appropriate strengths by adjusting diluent.

How to reconstitute

Follow the general guidelines described here when reconstituting a powder for injection.

Learn from the label

Begin by checking the label of the powder container. The label tells you the quantity of drug in a vial or ampule, the amount and type of diluent to add to the powder, and the strength and expiration date of the resulting solution.

Fluid out exceeds fluid in

When a diluent is added to a powder, the fluid volume increases. That's why the label calls for less diluent than the total volume of the prepared solution. For example, the instructions may say to add 1.7 ml of diluent to a vial of powdered drug to obtain 2 ml of prepared solution.

Check out the chambers

Some drugs that need reconstitution are packaged in vials with two chambers separated by a rubber stopper. The upper chamber contains the diluent, and the lower chamber contains the powdered drug. (See *Two chambers [one's a powder room!]*.)

When you depress the top of the vial, the stopper dislodges, allowing the diluent to flow into the lower chamber, where it can mix with the powdered drug. Then you can remove the correct amount of solution with a syringe.

Say it with an equation

To determine how much solution to give, refer to the drug label for information about the dose strength of the prepared solution. For example, to give 500 mg of a drug when the dose strength of the solution is 1 g (or 1,000 mg)/10 ml, set up a proportion with fractions as follows:

$$\frac{X}{500 \text{ mg}} = \frac{10 \text{ ml}}{1,000 \text{ mg}}$$

If information about a drug's dose strength isn't on the label, check the package insert. The label or insert will also list the type and amount of diluent needed, the dose strength after reconstitution, and special instructions about administration and storage after reconstitution. (See *Inspect the insert*, page 198.)

Two chambers (one's a powder room!)

Some drugs that require reconstitution are packaged in vials with two chambers separated by a rubber stopper. In the illustration below, note that the upper chamber contains the diluent and the lower chamber contains the powder. The plunger is depressed to inject the diluent into the powder.

— Plunger

— Diluent

— Rubber stopper

— Powder

Special considerations

When you reconstitute a powder that comes in multiple strengths, be especially careful in choosing the most appropriate strength for the prescribed dose. (See *One powder, three strengths*.)

Label logic

After you have reconstituted a drug, be sure you label it with the following information:
- your initials
- the reconstitution date
- the expiration date
- the dose strength.

Real world problems

The following problems show how to calculate the amount of reconstituted drug to give a patient.

Before you give that drug!

Inspect the insert

The package inserts that are included with drugs often provide a great deal of information that may not be on the outer label. For example, the drug label for ceftazidime provides no information about reconstitution, but the package insert does. These are the possible diluent combinations as they appear in the package insert that comes with this drug.

Vial size	Diluent to be added	Approximate available	Approximate average concentration
I.M. or I.V. direct (bolus) injection			
1 g	3.0 ml	3.6 ml	280 mg/ml
I.V. infusion			
1 g	10 ml	10.6 ml	95 mg/ml
2 g	10 ml	11.2 ml	180 mg/ml

Penicillin puzzler (the solution is in the solution)

The doctor prescribes *100,000 U of penicillin* for your patient, but the only available vial holds 1 million U. The drug label says to add 4.5 ml of normal saline solution to yield 1 million U/5 ml. How much solution should you administer after reconstitution?

Here's how to solve this problem using fractions:

• First, dilute the powder according to the instructions on the label. Then set up the first fraction with the known penicillin dose:

$$\frac{1,000,000 \text{ U}}{5 \text{ ml}}$$

Advice from the experts

One powder, three strengths

Many drugs are available in more than one strength. Here's one example:

Nafcillin sodium for injection comes in three dose strengths — 10 mg/ml, 20 mg/ml, and 50 mg/ml — as shown below. The availability of multiple strengths allows you to select the one that's most appropriate for your patient's needs.

Less is more

For example, if a patient who must restrict fluid intake needs to receive 1 g of nafcillin sodium, you should choose the 50 mg/ml dose strength because it requires less fluid to reconstitute. As the label states, obtaining this dose strength requires adding 20 ml of diluent during reconstitution. This gives you a concentration of 1 g in 20 ml. You can draw 20 ml of solution to administer the prescribed dose of 1 g.

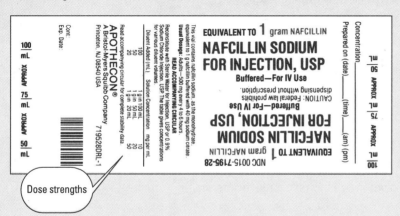

Dose strengths

• Set up the second fraction with the desired dose and the unknown amount of solution:

$$\frac{100,000 \text{ U}}{X}$$

• Put these fractions into a proportion:

$$\frac{1,000,000 \text{ U}}{5 \text{ ml}} = \frac{100,000 \text{ U}}{X}$$

• Cross-multiply the fractions:

$$5 \text{ ml} \times 100,000 \text{ U} = X \times 1,000,000 \text{ U}$$

• Solve for X by dividing each side of the equation by 1 million U and canceling units that appear in both the numerator and denominator:

$$\frac{5 \text{ ml} \times 100,000 \cancel{\text{U}}}{1,000,000 \cancel{\text{U}}} = \frac{X \text{ ml} \times \cancel{1,000,000 \text{ U}}}{\cancel{1,000,000 \text{ U}}}$$

$$X = \frac{500,000 \text{ ml}}{1,000,000}$$

$$X = 0.5 \text{ ml}$$

The amount of solution that yields 100,000 U of penicillin after reconstitution is 0.5 ml.

Deciphering diluents

Your patient needs 25 mg of gentamicin I.M. The label says to add 1.3 ml sterile diluent to yield 50 mg/1.5 ml. How many milliliters of reconstituted solution should you give the patient?

This is how to solve this problem using ratios:
• First, dilute the powder according to the instructions on the label. Then set up the first ratio with the known gentamicin dose:

$$50 \text{ mg} : 1.5 \text{ ml}$$

• Set up the second ratio with the desired dose and the unknown amount of solution:

$$25 \text{ mg} : X$$

• Put these ratios into a proportion:

$$50 \text{ mg} : 1.5 \text{ ml} :: 25 \text{ mg} : X$$

• Set up an equation by multiplying the means and the extremes:

$$1.5 \text{ ml} \times 25 \text{ mg} = X \times 50 \text{ mg}$$

• Solve for X. Divide each side of the equation by 50 mg and cancel units that appear in both the numerator and denominator:

$$\frac{1.5 \text{ ml} \times 25 \text{ mg}}{50 \text{ mg}} = \frac{X \times 50 \text{ mg}}{50 \text{ mg}}$$

$$X = \frac{37.5 \text{ ml}}{50}$$

$$X = 0.75 \text{ ml}$$

The patient should receive 0.75 ml of the solution.

Attaining the ampicillin answer

The doctor orders *500 mg of ampicillin* for your patient. A 1-g vial of powdered ampicillin is available. The label says to add 4.5 ml sterile water to yield 1 g/5 ml. How many milliliters of reconstituted ampicillin should you give?

Here's how to solve this problem using fractions:

• First, dilute the powder according to the instructions on the label. Then set up the first fraction with the known ampicillin dose (recall that 1 g equals 1,000 mg):

$$\frac{1,000 \text{ mg}}{5 \text{ ml}}$$

• Set up the second fraction with the desired dose and the unknown amount of solution:

$$\frac{500 \text{ mg}}{X}$$

• Put these fractions into a proportion, making sure the same units of measure appear in both numerators. In this case, the units must both be grams or milligrams. If you use milligrams, the proportion would be:

$$\frac{1,000 \text{ mg}}{5 \text{ ml}} = \frac{500 \text{ mg}}{X}$$

• Cross-multiply the fractions:

$$1,000 \text{ mg} \times X = 500 \text{ mg} \times 5 \text{ ml}$$

• Solve for X by dividing each side of the equation by 1,000 mg and canceling units that appear in both the numerator and denominator:

$$\frac{1,000 \text{ mg} \times X}{1,000 \text{ mg}} = \frac{500 \text{ mg} \times 5 \text{ ml}}{1,000 \text{ mg}}$$

$$X = \frac{2,500 \text{ ml}}{1,000}$$

$$X = 2.5 \text{ ml}$$

You should give the patient 2.5 ml of the solution, which will deliver 500 mg of ampicillin.

Quick quiz

1. To administer the medication in a prefilled syringe, you need:
    A.   a Carpuject or Tubex.
    B.   a standard syringe.
    C.   dead space.

Answer: A. Prefilled syringes come with a cartridge-needle unit and require a special holder called a Carpuject or Tubex to release the drug from the cartridge.

2. You need to purge a prefilled syringe before administering a drug because:
    A.   the cartridge won't work otherwise.
    B.   the syringe may contain air.
    C.   this ensures needle patency.

Answer: B. You must purge the air from a prefilled syringe. Because a small amount of drug is wasted during purging, most manufacturers add a little extra drug to prefilled syringes.

3. The only insulin that can be given I.V. is:
   A.   NPH.
   B.   lente.
   C.   regular.

Answer: C. Regular insulin can be given I.V. NPH and lente insulin must be given S.C.

4. The longest-acting insulin is:
   A.   regular.
   B.   lente.
   C.   ultralente.

Answer: C. Ultralente insulin has a duration of 36 hours. Regular insulin lasts 6 to 8 hours, and lente insulin lasts 18 to 24 hours.

5. The needle used for an intradermal injection is:
   A.   25G to 27G and $^3/_8''$ to $^5/_8''$ long.
   B.   14G to 18G and 1″ to $1^1/_2''$ long.
   C.   22G and $^3/_4''$ long.

Answer: A. A 1-ml syringe, calibrated in 0.01-ml increments, is usually used with this needle for an intradermal injection.

6. In an S.C. injection, the drug is injected into the:
   A.   tissue above the dermis.
   B.   tissue below the dermis.
   C.   tissue in the vastus lateralis.

Answer: B. An S.C. injection puts the drug into the subcutaneous tissue, located below the dermis but above the muscle.

7. A percentage solution can be expressed in terms of:
   A.   weight/volume and volume/volume.
   B.   weight/weight and volume/volume.
   C.   weight/weight and strength/volume.

Answer: A. Percentage solutions are expressed as weight/volume or volume/volume. These are the clearest and most common ways to label or describe solutions.

Wouldn't it be nice if you could just pull the correct answer out of a hat?

8.   When a diluent is added to a powder for injection, the fluid volume:

    A.   increases.

    B.   decreases.

    C.   stays the same.

Answer: A. When a diluent is added to a powder, the fluid volume increases. That's why the label calls for less diluent than the total volume of the prepared solution.

Scoring

☆☆☆   If you answered all eight items correctly, bravo! You've earned the right to say to anyone "this won't hurt a bit."

☆☆   If you answered six or seven correctly, you're almost a parenteral powerhouse!

☆   If you answered fewer than six correctly, okay! Remember the golden rule of dosage calculations: Keep things in proportion.

12

Calculating I.V. infusions

Just the facts

In this chapter, you'll learn:

♦ how to calculate drip rates and flow rates

♦ how to regulate an infusion manually and electronically

♦ how to calculate infusion time and regulate infusions

♦ how to calculate and monitor infusions of blood, total parenteral nutrition, heparin, insulin, and electrolytes.

A look at I.V. infusions

Careful administration of I.V. fluids is critical, especially when dealing with patients who are susceptible to fluid volume changes. Rapid infusion of I.V. fluids or blood products may seriously threaten your patient's health.

Work from the outside-in

To administer I.V. fluids safely, you need information specifying how much fluid to give, the correct length of time for administration, the type of fluid, and what may be added to the fluid. Start by examining the outside of a full I.V. bag and learn to identify all its components. (See *Read the bag*, page 206.)

Next, you'll need to be able to select the proper tubing, calculate drip rates and flow rates, and become comfortable working with I.V. equipment such as electronic infusion devices. (See *Checking an I.V.*, page 206.)

Before you give that drug!

Read the bag

The outside of an I.V. bag is an important source of information for calculating infusion rates and times. Read it carefully!

Total volume of I.V. bag

Name and concentration of I.V. fluid

Graduations for measuring

Advice from the experts

Checking an I.V.

You can save time by assessing your patient's I.V. infusion at the beginning of every shift. Performing checks early helps avoid confusion when your shift gets busy.

• Are the time, volume, and rate labeled correctly? If so, do they match the order?

• Check maintenance fluids and drug infusions, such as insulin, dopamine, and morphine. Are the additives correct? Are they in the right solutions?

• After calculating the drug dosage, check the bag again to verify that the solution is labeled with the time, name, and amount of drug added.

• If an electronic infusion device is being used, is it set correctly?

• Examine the tubing from the bag down to the patient to see if the drug is infusing into the correct I.V. port. This is critical when a patient has multiple lines.

Administering I.V. fluids

To safely and accurately administer I.V. fluids to your patient, you must select the proper tubing. Selection of I.V. tubing plays an important role in calculating I.V. infusion rates.

Most facilities stock I.V. tubing in two sizes: microdrip and macrodrip. Microdrip tubing, as its name implies, delivers smaller drops than macrodrip. Microdrip also delivers more drops per minute.

Targeting the right tube

To decide the right size tubing for your patient, you should first understand the purpose of the infusion and the desired infusion rate. If the infusion rate for a solution is relatively fast — for example, 125 ml/hour — select macrodrip tubing. If the infusion rate is relatively slow — for example, 40 ml/hour — select microdrip tubing. If you use macrodrip tubing for a slow infusion, maintaining accurate I.V. flow may be difficult if not impossible. (See *Tube tips*.)

Calculating drip rates

Your next step is to determine the number of drops of solution you want to infuse per minute. In other words, you want to determine a *drip rate*.

To calculate the drip rate, you need to know the calibration for the I.V. tubing you've selected. Different I.V. solution sets deliver fluids at varying amounts per drop. The *drip factor* refers to the number of drops per milliliter of solution calibrated for an administration set.

The drip factor is listed on the package containing the I.V. tubing administration set. For a standard (macrodrip) administration set, the drip factor usually is 10, 15, or 20 gtt/ml (drops per milliliter). For a microdrip (minidrip) set, it's 60 gtt/ml. (See *Quick drip rate guide*, page 208.)

Drip, drip, drip...

One way to calculate the drip rate is to use the formula below:

$$\text{Drip rate in drops/minute} = \frac{\text{Total milliliters}}{\text{Total minutes}} \times \text{Drip factor in drops/ml}$$

The three examples that follow show how to calculate the drip rate using this formula.

Drip rate difficulty

Your patient needs an infusion of D_5W at 125 ml/hour. If the tubing set is calibrated at 15 gtt/ml, what's the drip rate?
• First, convert 1 hour to 60 minutes to fit the formula.

Advice from the experts

Tube tips

Follow these rules when selecting I.V. tubing:
• Use macrodrip tubing for infusions of at least 80 ml/hour.
• Use microdrip tubing for infusions of less than 80 ml/hour and for pediatric patients (to prevent fluid overload).
• With electronic infusion devices, select the tubing specifically made to work with those devices.

Before you give that drug!

Quick drip rate guide

When calculating the drip rate of I.V. solutions, remember that the number of drops required to deliver 1 ml varies with the type of administration set and the manufacturer. To calculate the drip rate, you need to know the drip factor for each product. As a quick reference, consult the table below.

Manufacturer	Drip factor	Drops/minute to infuse (drip rate)					
		500 ml/24 hr	1,000 ml/24 hr	1,000 ml/20 hr	1,000 ml/10 hr	1,000 ml/8 hr	1,000 ml/6 hr
		21 ml/hr	42 ml/hr	50 ml/hr	100 ml/hr	125 ml/hr	166 ml/hr
Abbott	15 gtt/ml	5 gtt	10 gtt	12 gtt	25 gtt	31 gtt	42 gtt
Baxter-Healthcare	10 gtt/ml	3 gtt	7 gtt	8 gtt	17 gtt	21 gtt	28 gtt
Cutter	20 gtt/ml	7 gtt	14 gtt	17 gtt	34 gtt	42 gtt	56 gtt
IVAC	20 gtt/ml	7 gtt	14 gtt	17 gtt	34 gtt	42 gtt	56 gtt
McGaw	15 gtt/ml	5 gtt	10 gtt	12 gtt	25 gtt	31 gtt	42 gtt

• Then set up a fraction. Place the volume of the infusion in the numerator. Place the number of minutes in which the volume is to be infused as the denominator:

$$\frac{125 \text{ ml}}{60 \text{ minutes}}$$

• To determine X — or the number of drops per minute to be infused — multiply the fraction by the drip factor. Cancel units that appear in both the numerator and denominator:

$$X = \frac{125 \text{ ml}}{60 \text{ minutes}} \times \frac{15 \text{ gtt}}{\text{ml}}$$

• Solve for X by dividing the numerator by the denominator:

$$X = \frac{125 \times 15 \text{ gtt}}{60 \text{ minutes}}$$

$$X = \frac{1,875 \text{ gtt}}{60 \text{ minutes}}$$

$$X = 31.25 \text{ gtt/minute}$$

The drip rate is 31.25 gtt/minute, rounded to 31 gtt/minute.

Cheat sheet

Drip rate

• Number of drops infused per minute
• Formula — total milliliters ÷ total minutes × drip factor in gtt/ml
• Drip factor — number of drops per ml of solution that the I.V. tubing is designed to deliver

To determine the drip rate, I need to know the drip factor!

What a drip!

You receive an order that reads *KCl 40 mEq in 100 ml NS over 40 minutes.* You decide to use a controller for the infusion, along with a tubing set calibrated at 60 gtt/ml.

What's the drip rate?
• Set up the fraction. Place the volume of the infusion in the numerator. Place the number of minutes for the infusion in the denominator:

$$\frac{100 \text{ ml}}{40 \text{ minutes}}$$

• To determine the number of drops per minute to be infused (solve for X), multiply the fraction by the drip factor. Cancel units that appear in both the numerator and denominator:

$$X = \frac{100 \text{ ml}}{40 \text{ minutes}} \times \frac{60 \text{ gtt}}{\text{ml}}$$

• To solve for X, divide the numerator by the denominator:

$$X = \frac{100 \times 60 \text{ gtt}}{40 \text{ minutes}}$$

$$X = \frac{6,000 \text{ gtt}}{40 \text{ minutes}}$$

$$X = 150 \text{ gtt/minute}$$

The drip rate is 150 gtt/minute.

Drip rate drill

Your patient needs 15 ml of erythromycin, which is equal to 500 mg. The infusion is to be completed in 30 minutes using a tubing set calibrated to 20 gtt/ml.

What's the drip rate?
• Set up a fraction. Place the volume of the infusion in the numerator. Place the number of minutes in which the volume is to be infused in the denominator:

$$\frac{15 \text{ ml}}{30 \text{ minutes}}$$

• Multiply the fraction by the drip factor to determine the number of drops per minute to be infused (solve for X). Cancel the units of measure that appear in both the numerator and denominator:

$$X = \frac{15 \text{ ml}}{30 \text{ minutes}} \times \frac{20 \text{ gtt}}{\text{ml}}$$

- Solve for X by dividing the numerator by the denominator:

$$X = \frac{15 \times 20 \text{ gtt}}{30 \text{ minutes}}$$

$$X = \frac{300 \text{ gtt}}{30 \text{ minutes}}$$

$$X = 10 \text{ gtt/minute}$$

The drip rate is 10 gtt/minute.

To determine the flow rate, I need to know the total volume and the amount of time for the infusion.

Calculating the flow rate

If your patient is receiving a large-volume infusion to maintain hydration or to replace fluids or electrolytes, you may need to calculate the flow rate. The *flow rate* is the number of milliliters of fluid to administer over 1 hour. To perform this calculation, you need to know the total volume to be infused in milliliters and the amount of time for the infusion.

Use this formula:

$$\text{Flow rate} = \frac{\text{total volume ordered}}{\text{number of hours}}$$

For example, if your patient needs 1,000 ml of fluid over 8 hours, find the flow rate by dividing the volume by the number of hours:

$$\text{Flow rate} = \frac{1,000 \text{ ml}}{8 \text{ hours}} = 125 \text{ ml/hour}$$

The flow rate is 125 ml/hour.

Time it for 2 hours

Here's another example: Your patient needs 250 ml of normal saline solution over 2 hours.

What's the infusion rate?

- First, set up the equation. Then divide 250 ml by 2 hours to find the flow rate in milliliters per hour:

$$\text{Flow rate} = \frac{250 \text{ ml}}{2 \text{ hours}} = 125 \text{ ml/hour}$$

The flow rate is 125 ml/hour.

Cheat sheet

Flow rate

- The number of milliliters of fluid administered over 1 hour
- Formula—total volume ordered ÷ number of hours

Quick calculation of drip rates

Here's a shortcut for calculating I.V. drip rates. It's based on the fact that all drip factors can be evenly divided into 60.

For macrodrip sets, use these rules to calculate drip rates:
- For sets that deliver 10 gtt/ml, divide the flow rate by 6.
- For sets that deliver 15 gtt/ml, divide the flow rate by 4.
- For sets that deliver 20 gtt/ml, divide the flow rate by 3.

With a microdrip set (drip factor of 60 gtt/ml), simply remember that the drip rate is the same as the flow rate.

Why the microdrip flow rate equals the drip rate

Here is the equation for determining drip rate for a solution with a flow rate of 125 ml/hour (125 ml/60 minutes) when using a microdrip set (drip factor of 60 gtt/ml). Note that the number of minutes and the number of drops per milliliter cancel each other out.

Multiply the flow rate by the drip factor...

$$\text{Drip rate} = \frac{125 \text{ ml}}{60 \text{ minutes}} \times \frac{60 \text{ gtt}}{1 \text{ ml}}$$

$$\text{Drip rate} = 125 \text{ gtt/minute}$$

...to find the drip rate.

The drip rate (125 gtt/minute) is the same as the number of milliliters of fluid per hour (flow rate).

Take the shortcut

The doctor prescribes *1,000 ml of normal saline to be infused over 12 hours.* If your administration set delivers 15 gtt/ml, what's the drip rate?
- First, determine the flow rate *(X)* by dividing the number of milliliters to be delivered by the number of hours:

$$X = \frac{1,000 \text{ ml}}{12 \text{ hours}} = 83.3 \text{ ml/hour}$$

- Remember the rule: For sets that deliver 15 gtt/ml, divide the flow rate by 4 to determine the drip rate.
- Next, set up an equation to determine the drip rate which now becomes *X* and solve for *X*. Divide the flow rate by 4:

$$X = \frac{83.3}{4}$$

$$X = 20.8 \text{ gtt/minute}$$

The drip rate is 20.8 gtt/minute, rounded to 21 gtt/minute.

Follow the golden microdrip rule

See if you can solve the following problem without pencil, paper, or calculator:

Your patient is to receive an I.V. infusion of 150 ml/hour using a 60 gtt/ml set. What's the drip rate?

First, determine the flow rate. Recall that the flow rate is the number of milliliters of fluid to administer over 1 hour. Simply from reading the problem we see that the flow rate is 150 ml/hr.

Now remember the rule: With a microdrip set, the drip rate is the same as the flow rate. Thus, the drip rate is 150 gtt/minute. Just think: You're doing dosage calculations without any math!

150 ml/hour equals 150 gtt/minute. Now that's the kind of math I like!

Calculating infusion time

When you can calculate the flow rate and drip rate, you're ready to compute the time required for infusion of a specified volume of I.V. fluid. This calculation will help you keep the infusion on schedule and start the next infusion on time. It also will help you perform laboratory tests, such as the chemistry and electrolyte assessments that commonly accompany infusions, on time.

To calculate the infusion time, you must know the flow rate in milliliters per hour and the volume to be infused. Here's the formula:

$$\text{Infusion time} = \frac{\text{volume to be infused}}{\text{flow rate}}$$

The examples below show how to use this formula to calculate infusion times.

Be back in _____ minutes!

If you plan to infuse 1 L of D_5W at 50 ml/hour, what's the infusion time?
• First, convert 1 L to 1,000 ml to make units of measure that are equivalent.
• Then set up the fraction with the volume of the infusion as the numerator and the flow rate as the denominator:

$$\frac{1,000 \text{ ml}}{50 \text{ ml/hour}}$$

• Next, solve for X by dividing 1,000 by 50 and canceling units that appear in both the numerator and denominator:

$$X = \frac{1,000 \text{ ml}}{50 \text{ ml/hour}}$$

$$X = 20 \text{ hours}$$

The D_5W will infuse in 20 hours.

The bag will be empty at _____ o'clock

Your patient requires 500 ml of normal saline solution at 80 ml/hour. What's the infusion time? If the normal saline solution is hung at 5 a.m., what time will the infusion end?
- Set up a fraction. Place the volume of the infusion as the numerator and the flow rate as the denominator:

$$X = \frac{500 \text{ ml}}{80 \text{ ml/hour}}$$

- Solve for X by dividing 500 by 80 and canceling units that appear in both the numerator and denominator:

$$X = \frac{500 \cancel{\text{ml}}}{80 \cancel{\text{ml}}/\text{hour}}$$

$$X = 6.25 \text{ hours}$$

The normal saline solution will infuse in 6.25 hours, which means that the bag will be empty at 11:15 a.m.

Keep the infusion on schedule. Know your formula!

An alternative formula

Suppose all you know are the volume to be infused, the drip rate, and the drip factor. Then use the alternative formula here to calculate the infusion time:

$$\text{Infusion time in hours} = \frac{\text{volume to be infused}}{(\text{drip rate/drip factor}) \times 60 \text{ minutes}}$$

A saline solution (literally)

A doctor prescribes *250 ml of normal saline I.V. at 32 gtt/minute*. The drip factor is 15 gtt/ml. What's the infusion time?
- Set up the formula with the known information:

$$\text{Infusion time} = \frac{250 \text{ ml}}{(32 \text{ gtt/minute}/15 \text{ gtt/ml}) \times 60 \text{ minutes}}$$

- Divide the drip rate by the drip factor. (Remember, to *divide* a complex fraction, multiply the dividend by the reciprocal of the divisor.) Cancel units that appear in both the numerator and denominator:

$$\frac{32 \cancel{\text{gtt}}/\text{minute}}{15 \cancel{\text{gtt}}/\text{ml}} = 2.13 \text{ ml/minute}$$

- Rewrite the equation (solve for X) with the result (2.13 ml/minute) placed in the denominator. Cancel units that appear in both the numerator and denominator:

Cheat sheet

Infusion time

- Method #1: infusion time = infused volume ÷ flow rate
- Method #2: infusion time = infused volume ÷ drip rate/drip factor × 60 minutes

$$X = \frac{250 \text{ ml}}{(2.13 \text{ ml/minute}) \times 60 \text{ minutes}}$$

- To find the infusion time, solve for X:

$$X = \frac{250}{2.13 \times 60}$$

$$X = \frac{250}{127.8}$$

- Round off the denominator, and then divide it into the numerator:

$$X = \frac{250}{128}$$

$$X = 1.95 \text{ hours}$$

- The infusion time is 1.95 hours. Convert the decimal fraction portion of this time to minutes by multiplying by 60:

$$0.95 \text{ hour} \times 60 \text{ minutes} = 57 \text{ minutes}$$

The infusion time is 1 hour and 57 minutes.

Heads-up! Here comes Hespan...

If 500 ml of hetastarch (Hespan) are infusing at 40 gtt/minute with a set calibration of 20 gtt/ml, what's the infusion time?
- Use the information you know to set up a formula:

$$X = \frac{500 \text{ ml}}{(40 \text{ gtt/minute/20 gtt/ml}) \times 60 \text{ minutes}}$$

- Divide the drip rate by the drip factor. Cancel units that appear in both the numerator and denominator:

$$\frac{40 \text{ gtt/minute}}{20 \text{ gtt/ml}} = 2 \text{ ml/minute}$$

- Rewrite the equation (solving for X) with the new denominator (2 ml/minute). Cancel units that appear in both the numerator and denominator:

$$X = \frac{500 \text{ ml}}{(2 \text{ ml/minute}) \times 60 \text{ minutes}}$$

- To find the infusion time, solve for X:

$$X = \frac{500}{2 \times 60}$$

$$X = \frac{500}{120}$$

- Divide the numerator by the denominator:

$$X = 4.166 = 4.17$$

- The infusion time is 4.166 hours, which rounds off to 4.17 hours. To convert the decimal fraction to minutes, multiply by 60 and then round off the number:

$$0.17 \text{ hour} \times 60 \text{ minutes} = 10.2 \text{ minutes} = 10 \text{ minutes}$$

The infusion time is 4 hours and 10 minutes.

This should Ringer bell

If you infuse 1,050 ml of lactated Ringer's solution at 25 gtt/minute using a set calibration of 10 gtt/ml, what's the infusion time?
- Use the information you know to set up the formula:

$$X = \frac{1,050 \text{ ml}}{(25 \text{ gtt/minute/10 gtt/ml}) \times 60 \text{ minutes}}$$

- Divide the drip rate by the drip factor. Cancel units that appear in both the numerator and denominator:

$$\frac{25 \text{ gtt/minute}}{10 \text{ gtt/ml}} = 2.5 \text{ ml/minute}$$

- Rewrite the equation (solving for X) using the result (2.5 ml/minute) in the denominator. Cancel units that appear in both the numerator and denominator:

$$X = \frac{1,050 \text{ ml}}{(2.5 \text{ ml/minute}) \times 60 \text{ minutes}}$$

- To find the infusion time, solve for X:

$$X = \frac{1,050}{2.5 \times 60}$$

$$X = \frac{1,050}{150}$$

- Divide the numerator by the denominator:

$$X = 7 \text{ hours}$$

The infusion time is 7 hours.

Let's see, 1,050 ml of lactated Ringer's... well, I'll have to divide the drip rate by the drip factor.

Regulating infusions

After you start an infusion, you must be careful to regulate the I.V. flow. You can do this:
- manually
- using a pump
- using a patient-controlled analgesia (PCA) pump.

Regulating I.V. flow manually

To manually regulate the I.V. flow, count the number of drops going into the drip chamber. While counting the drops, adjust the flow with the roller clamp until the fluid is infusing at the appropriate number of drops per minute.

Fifteen seconds works fine

To save time, don't count for a full minute — calculate the drip rate for 15 seconds only. To do this, divide the prescribed drip rate by 4 (because 15 seconds is $\frac{1}{4}$ of a minute). For example, if the prescribed drip rate is 31 gtt/minute, divide 31 by 4 to get 8 (round 31 up to 32 first so it will divide evenly). Then adjust the roller clamp until the drip chamber shows 8 drops in 15 seconds.

Afterward, time-tape the I.V. bag to ensure that the solution is given at the prescribed rate and to make recording fluid intake easier. (See *Taped up and ready to drip.*)

Electronic infusion pumps

Electronic infusion pumps facilitate I.V. administration. Pumps administer fluid under positive pressure and are calibrated by drip rate and volume.

Steady as she goes

When using a pump, set the device to deliver a constant amount of solution per hour, following the manufacturer's directions.

The electronic edge

Electronic infusion pumps offer many advantages, such as:
- allowing you to easily control the rate, or volume, by setting it on the machine
- shortening the time needed to calculate an infusion rate
- requiring less maintenance than standard devices that drip fluid by gravity
- providing greater accuracy than standard devices.

Save yourself time. Calculate the drip rate for 15 seconds instead of for a full minute. Divide by four.

Advice from the experts

Taped up and ready to drip

Time-taping an I.V. bag helps ensure that an I.V. solution is administered at the prescribed rate. It also helps facilitate recording of fluid intake.

To time-tape an I.V. bag, place a strip of adhesive tape from the top to the bottom of the bag, next to the fluid level markings. (This illustration shows a bag time-taped for a rate of 100 ml/hour beginning at 10 a.m.)

0 marks the spot.

Next to the "0" marking, record the time that you hung the bag. Then, knowing the hourly rate, mark each hour on the tape next to the corresponding fluid marking. At the bottom of the tape, mark the time at which the solution will be completely infused.

Ink alert

Don't write directly on the bag with a felt tip marker because the ink may seep into the fluid. Some manufacturers provide printed time-tapes for use with their solutions.

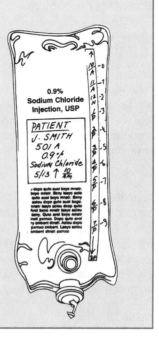

Special features

Some pumps keep track of the amount of fluid that has been infused, helping maintain accurate intake and output records. Many have alarms that signal when the fluid container is empty or when a mechanical problem occurs. Some devices have variable pressure limits that prevent them from pumping fluids into infiltrated sites.

Regulating I.V. flow with pumps

When using a pump to regulate I.V. flow, program the device based on your calculation of the infusion rate. Remember that infusion pumps can make mistakes — they don't eliminate the need for careful calculations and assessment of infusion rates over time. So check the infusion by counting the drips in the chamber just as you would with manual regulation.

Programming the pump

To determine the pump settings, consider the volume of fluid to be given and the total infusion time. With most devices, you'll need to program both the amount of fluid to be infused and the hourly flow rate. However, some devices require you to program the flow rate per minute or the drip rate.

Patient-controlled analgesia pumps

One popular infusion device is the computerized PCA pump, which allows a patient to self-administer an analgesic by pushing a button. You program the pump to deliver a precise dose every time. The pump also can be programmed to deliver a basal dose of drug in addition to the patient-controlled dose. (See *Putting your patient in control.*)

Leveling blood levels

PCA pumps keep blood concentrations of analgesics consistent. With the traditional approach — giving an intramuscular analgesic every few hours — blood levels fluctuate, so patients have periods of heavy sedation alternating with periods of increasing pain.

Two added benefits of PCA pumps are that patients tend to take less medication than they do with the traditional approach and also develop a greater feeling of control over their pain.

Pump-provided protection

Several safety features are built into PCA pumps. Drug dose and administration frequency are programmed, preventing the patient from medicating himself too often. If the patient tries to overmedicate, the machine simply ignores the request.

Also, some pumps record both the number of requests and the number of times the patient actually receives medication. This lets you evaluate whether the doctor needs to increase or decrease the drug dose.

PCA password

PCA pumps require you to use an access code or key before entering drug dose and frequency information into the system. This prevents unauthorized people from tampering with or accidentally resetting the pump. Some machines even record unauthorized entries.

PCA prep parameters

When preparing a PCA pump for a patient, follow these guidelines:

• Draw the correct amount and concentration of drug—usually morphine—and insert it into the PCA pump. Prefilled cartridges are usually available.
• Program the pump according to the manufacturer's directions.
• Carefully read the PCA log, and then record the information based on your facility's policy. A typical order might state the following: *Start MSO$_4$ PCA. Give 2 mg/hr basal rate and 1 mg/q15 min on demand, with a lock-out of 6 mg/4 hr.*

Recording drug dosage with a PCA

When interpreting the PCA log, note the strength (number of milligrams per milliliter) of drug solution in the syringe. You'll need this information to calculate the dose received by the patient.

Covering the basals

Also note the number of times the patient received the drug throughout the time covered by your assessment (usually over 4 hours). If your patient is receiving a basal dose, note that as well.

Advice from the experts

Putting your patient in control

A computerized patient-controlled analgesia (PCA) pump, such as that shown to the right, allows your patient to give himself pain medication with the push of a button. With PCA pumps, patients tend to use less medication than they do with the traditional approach and also develop a greater feeling of control over their pain.

By multiplying the number of injections by the volume of each injection and adding the basal dose, you can determine the amount of solution the patient received.

Multiply this amount by the solution strength to find the total amount of drug, as shown in this equation:

Fluid volume × solution strength = total medication received

Record this amount in milligrams in the patient's medication record.

Promoting PCA precision

Most facilities require the nurse who prepares the syringe to record the amount of fluid and drug in the syringe. Each nurse who checks the PCA log double-checks and records this information. The record enables you to double-check the accuracy of everyone's calculations.

Adjusting the infusion rate

No matter how carefully you calculate the drip rate and adjust the flow rate of an I.V. infusion, the rate still may change. Why? Perhaps the patient changed position, the I.V. tubing became kinked, or the I.V. infiltrated. Such factors cause the infusion to run ahead or behind schedule.

Don't hesitate to recalculate

When problems occur, recalculate the drip rate taking into account the remaining time and volume. If the fluid has infused too slowly, see if the patient can tolerate an increased rate by checking his cardiac and respiratory status. Look for a history of renal insufficiency, pulmonary edema, or any other condition that increases the risk of fluid overload.

If I.V. fluid has infused too quickly, slow or stop the infusion and assess for signs of fluid overload, such as crackles and increased blood pressure. Call the doctor if these occur.

Are you up for a fluid challenge?

You may also need to adjust the infusion rate to perform a *fluid challenge*, the protocol for monitoring how a patient tolerates increased fluids. The fastest way to do a fluid challenge is by increasing the I.V. flow rate for a specified time and then reducing it to a maintenance rate. *However, be sure to use a fluid bolus cautiously in pediatric and geriatric patients.*

Cheat sheet

PCA log notes

- The strength of drug solution in syringe
- Number of drug administrations during assessment period
- Basal dose patient received, if any
- Amount of solution received = (number of injections × volume of injections + basal doses)
- Total amount of drug received = (amount of solution × solution strength)

Heparin and insulin infusions

The doctor may prescribe heparin or insulin to be added to a large-volume I.V. infusion. These drugs may be ordered in milliliters per hour, milligrams per hour, or units per hour. To administer them safely, you must calculate the drug dose so that it falls within therapeutic limits.

Calculating heparin doses

A common anticoagulant, heparin prevents the formation of new clots and slows the development of preexisting clots. Usually given by the I.V. route, it's ordered in doses of units per hour or milliliters per hour. Each dose is individualized based on the patient's coagulation status, which is measured by the partial thromboplastin time.

Flow rate

Accurately calculating the flow rate ensures that the heparin dose falls within safe and therapeutic limits. This type of calculation differs from the flow rate calculations discussed earlier because it's used to administer a drug, not just a fluid.

To calculate the hourly heparin flow rate, first determine the solution's concentration by dividing the units of drug added to the bag by the number of milliliters of solution. Then write a fraction stating the desired dose of heparin over the unknown flow rate. Then simply cross-multiply to find the unknown flow rate.

Here are some examples using simple proportions to find the solution.

Go with the flow! Calculate milliliters per hour.

An order states *heparin 40,000 U in 1 L of D_5W I.V. Infuse at 1,000 U/hr*. What's the flow rate in milliliters per hour?

• First, convert 1 L to 1,000 ml. Then write a fraction to express the known solution strength (units of drug divided by milliliters of solution):

$$\frac{40,000 \text{ U}}{1,000 \text{ ml}}$$

• Write a second fraction with the desired dose of heparin in the numerator and the unknown flow rate in the denominator:

$$\frac{1,000 \text{ U/hour}}{X}$$

When infusing heparin, you need to go with the flow.

- Put these fractions into a proportion:

$$\frac{40,000 \text{ U}}{1,000 \text{ ml}} = \frac{1,000 \text{ U/hour}}{X}$$

- To find the flow rate, solve for X by cross-multiplying:

$$40,000 \text{ U} \times X = 1,000 \text{ U/hour} \times 1,000 \text{ ml}$$

- Divide each side of the equation by 40,000 U and cancel units that appear in both the numerator and denominator:

$$\frac{40,000 \cancel{\text{U}} \times X}{40,000 \cancel{\text{U}}} = \frac{1,000 \cancel{\text{U}}/\text{hour} \times 1,000 \text{ ml}}{40,000 \cancel{\text{U}}}$$

$$X = \frac{1,000,000 \text{ ml/hour}}{40,000}$$

$$X = 25 \text{ ml/hour}$$

To administer heparin at 1,000 U/hour, you should set the flow rate at 25 ml/hour.

Heparin flow rate formula

- Determine solution's concentration: Divide units of drug added by the amount of solution in milliliters.
- State as a fraction: the desired dose over the unknown flow rate.
- Cross-multiply.

Know this flow?

You're about to administer a continuous infusion of 25,000 U of heparin in 250 ml of D_5W. If the patient is to receive 600 U/hour, what's the flow rate?

- Write a ratio to express the known solution strength (units of drug to milliliters of solution):

$$25,000 \text{ U} : 250 \text{ ml}$$

- Write a second ratio to describe the desired dose of heparin in relation to the unknown flow rate:

$$600 \text{ U/hour} : X$$

- Put these ratios into a proportion:

$$25,000 \text{ U} : 250 \text{ ml} :: 600 \text{ U/hour} : X$$

- Solve for X by multiplying the extremes and the means:

$$25,000 \text{ U} \times X = 600 \text{ U/hour} \times 250 \text{ ml}$$

- Divide each side of the equation by 25,000 U and cancel units that appear in both the numerator and denominator:

$$\frac{25,000 \cancel{\text{U}} \times X}{25,000 \cancel{\text{U}}} = \frac{600 \cancel{\text{U}}/\text{hour} \times 250 \text{ ml}}{25,000 \cancel{\text{U}}}$$

$$X = \frac{600 \times 250 \text{ ml/hour}}{25,000}$$

$$X = \frac{150,000 \text{ ml/hour}}{25,000}$$

$$X = 6 \text{ ml/hour}$$

To administer 600 U/hour, you should set the flow rate at 6 ml/hour.

Units per hour

If a heparin infusion is ordered in milliliters per hour, you may want to calculate it in units per hour, too. This determines the patient's drug dose so you can be sure it falls within a safe and therapeutic range.

Here's an example calculating units per hour.

You use units? Yes, units are useful.

A patient is receiving 20,000 U of heparin in 1,000 ml of D_5W I.V. at 30 ml/hour. What heparin dose is he receiving?

• Write a fraction to describe the known solution strength (units of drug divided by milliliters of solution):

$$\frac{20,000 \text{ U}}{1,000 \text{ ml}}$$

• Set up the second fraction with the flow rate in the denominator and the unknown dose of heparin in the numerator:

$$\frac{X}{30 \text{ ml/hour}}$$

• Write these fractions into a proportion:

$$\frac{20,000 \text{ U}}{1,000 \text{ ml}} = \frac{X}{30 \text{ ml/hour}}$$

• Solve for X by cross-multiplying:

$$1,000 \text{ ml} \times X = 30 \text{ ml/hour} \times 20,000 \text{ U}$$

• Divide each side of the equation by 1,000 ml and cancel units that appear in both the numerator and denominator:

$$\frac{\cancel{1,000 \text{ ml}} \times X}{\cancel{1,000 \text{ ml}}} = \frac{30 \cancel{\text{ ml}}\text{/hour} \times 20,000 \text{ U}}{1,000 \cancel{\text{ ml}}}$$

$$X = \frac{30 \times 20,000 \text{ U/hour}}{1,000}$$

$$X = \frac{600{,}000 \text{ U/hour}}{1{,}000}$$

$$X = 600 \text{ U/hour}$$

With the flow rate set at 30 ml/hour, the patient is receiving 600 U/hour of heparin.

Calculating continuous insulin infusions

An acutely ill diabetic patient may need to receive insulin by continuous infusion. This allows close control of insulin administration based on serial measurements of blood glucose levels.

You'll use an infusion pump to administer I.V. insulin. Regular insulin is the only type that can be administered by the I.V. route because it has a shorter duration of action than other insulins.

Insulin is usually prescribed in units per hour, but it may be ordered in milliliters per hour. In either case, the infusion should be in a concentration of 1 U/ml to avoid calculation errors that may have serious consequences. The examples here are based on common patient situations.

Insulin inquiry #1

Your patient needs a continuous infusion of 150 U of regular insulin in 150 ml of normal saline at 6 U/hour. What's the flow rate?
• Write a fraction to describe the known solution strength (units of drug over milliliters of solution):

$$\frac{150 \text{ U}}{150 \text{ ml}}$$

• Write a second fraction with the infusion rate in the numerator and the unknown flow rate in the denominator:

$$\frac{6 \text{ U/hour}}{X}$$

• Write the two fractions as a proportion:

$$\frac{150 \text{ U}}{150 \text{ ml}} = \frac{6 \text{ U/hour}}{X}$$

• Solve for X by cross-multiplying:

$$150 \text{ U} \times X = 6 \text{ U/hour} \times 150 \text{ ml}$$

• Divide each side of the equation by 150 U and cancel units that appear in both the numerator and denominator:

Doing all these calculations, you probably feel like you need an infusion of energy. Review your formulas!

$$\frac{\cancel{150\,U} \times X}{\cancel{150\,U}} = \frac{6\,U/\text{hour} \times \cancel{150}\,ml}{\cancel{150\,U}}$$

$$X = 6\text{ ml/hour}$$

To administer 6 U/hour of the prescribed insulin, you set the infusion pump's flow rate at 6 ml/hour.

Insulin inquiry #2

Your patient is receiving a continuous infusion of 50 U of regular insulin in 100 ml of normal saline at 10 ml/hour. How many units per hour is your patient receiving?
• Write a ratio to describe the known solution strength (units of insulin to milliliters of solution):

$$50\text{ U} : 100\text{ ml}$$

• Set up a second ratio comparing the unknown amount of insulin to the prescribed infusion rate:

$$X : 10\text{ ml/hour}$$

• Put these ratios into a proportion:

$$50\text{ U} : 100\text{ ml} :: X : 10\text{ ml/hour}$$

• Solve for X by multiplying the means and the extremes:

$$X \times 100\text{ ml} = 50\text{ U} \times 10\text{ ml/hour}$$

• Divide each side of the equation by 100 ml and cancel units that appear in both the numerator and denominator:

$$\frac{X \times \cancel{100\,ml}}{\cancel{100\,ml}} = \frac{50\text{ U} \times 10\,\cancel{ml}/\text{hour}}{100\,\cancel{ml}}$$

$$X = \frac{50\text{ U} \times 10/\text{hour}}{100}$$

$$X = \frac{500\text{ U/hour}}{100}$$

$$X = 5\text{ U/hour}$$

When the insulin infusion runs at 10 ml/hour, the patient receives 5 U/hour.

Cheat sheet

Insulin infusions

• Regular insulin is the only type administered by I.V. route.
• Use an infusion pump.
• Use concentrations of 1 U/ml.

Electrolyte and nutrient infusions

> You have to prepare and serve the correct amount of I.V. fluids to your patient.

I.V. fluids can be used to deliver electrolytes and nutrients directly into the patient's bloodstream.

Adding up the additives

Large-volume infusions with additives maintain or restore hydration or electrolyte status or supply additional electrolytes, vitamins, or other nutrients. In such cases, you may have to calculate and prepare the correct amount and add it to the solution.

Common additives include potassium chloride, vitamins B and C, and trace elements. Electrolytes may also be given in small-volume, intermittent infusions piggybacked into existing I.V. lines. (See *Calculating piggyback infusions.*)

Sometimes, you may need to combine more than one additive into a solution. Before calculating the correct amounts of each substance to inject, check the compatibility chart or consult the pharmacist to be sure that the additives can be mixed safely.

Prepare to prepare

If the additive isn't prepackaged in solution, either by the manufacturer or by the pharmacy, you must prepare the correct amount and add it to the solution. Then you must calculate the flow rate and the drip rate. To calculate the amount of additive, use the proportion method as you would for any prepared liquid drug. Here's an example.

Thinking about thiamine

Your patient requires 1,000 ml of D_5W with 150 mg of thiamine/L over 12 hours. The thiamine is available in a prepared syringe of 100 mg/ml. How many milliliters of thiamine must be added to the solution? What's the flow rate?
• Write the first ratio to describe the known solution strength (amount of drug per 1 ml):

$$100 \text{ mg} : 1 \text{ ml}$$

• Set up the second ratio. Write the amount of thiamine ordered on one side and the unknown amount to be added to the solution on the other side:

$$150 \text{ mg} : X$$

• Put these ratios into a proportion:

$$100 \text{ mg} : 1 \text{ ml} :: 150 \text{ mg} : X$$

- Solve for X by multiplying the extremes and the means:

$$X \times 100 \text{ mg} = 150 \text{ mg} \times 1 \text{ ml}$$

Peak technique

Calculating piggyback infusions

An I.V. piggyback is a small-volume, intermittent infusion that's connected to an existing I.V. line containing maintenance fluid. Most piggybacks contain antibiotics or electrolytes.

To calculate piggyback infusions, use proportions.

Piggyback problem
You receive an order for 500 mg of imipenem in 100 ml of normal saline solution to be infused over 1 hour. The imipenem vial contains 1,000 mg (1 g). The insert says to reconstitute the powder with 5 ml of normal saline solution. How much solution should you draw? What's the flow rate?

Solution solution
- Write the first ratio to describe the known solution strength (amount of drug compared to the known amount of solution):

$$1,000 \text{ mg} : 5 \text{ ml}$$

- Write the second ratio, which compares the desired dose of imipenem and the unknown amount of solution:

$$500 \text{ mg} : X$$

- Put these ratios into a proportion:

$$1,000 \text{ mg} : 5 \text{ ml} :: 500 \text{ mg} : X$$

- Multiply the extremes and the means:

$$1,000 \text{ mg} \times X = 500 \text{ mg} \times 5 \text{ ml}$$

- Solve for X by dividing each side of the equation by 1,000 mg and canceling units that appear in both the numerator and denominator:

$$\frac{1,000 \text{ mg} \times X}{1,000 \text{ mg}} = \frac{500 \text{ mg} \times 5 \text{ ml}}{1,000 \text{ mg}}$$

$$X = \frac{500 \times 5 \text{ ml}}{1,000}$$

$$X = \frac{2,500 \text{ ml}}{1,000}$$

$$X = 2.5 \text{ ml}$$

You should draw 2.5 ml of solution to get 500 mg of imipenem.

Flow rate
Recall that the flow rate is the number of milliliters of fluid to administer over 1 hour. So, in this case, the flow rate is 100 ml/hour.

Compatibility counts
After you've calculated an I.V. piggyback dose, make sure that the drugs to be infused together are compatible. The same goes for drugs mixed in the same syringe or I.V. bag. Drug compatibility charts can be time-savers — you should have one hanging in your unit's medication room. If not, use a drug handbook that includes a compatibility chart.

• Divide each side of the equation by 100 mg and cancel units that appear in both the numerator and denominator:

$$\frac{X \times \cancel{100 \text{ mg}}}{\cancel{100 \text{ mg}}} = \frac{150 \cancel{\text{ mg}} \times 1 \text{ ml}}{100 \cancel{\text{ mg}}}$$

$$X = \frac{150 \text{ ml}}{100}$$

$$X = 1.5 \text{ ml}$$

• You must add 1.5 ml of thiamine to the solution. If the flow rate is 1,000 ml over 12 hours, divide 1,000 by 12 to find the flow rate for 1 hour:

$$\frac{1,000 \text{ ml}}{12 \text{ hr}} = 83.3 \text{ ml/hr}$$

The flow rate is 83 ml/hour.

Blood and blood product infusions

The volume of fluid to be infused and the drip factor can be used for calculating transfusions of blood and blood products. During such transfusions, take care to prevent cell damage and ensure an adequate blood flow by using a special administration set that contains filters to remove agglutinated cells. The drip factor for these sets is usually 10 to 15 gtt/ml.

Generally, you'll use an 18G or larger I.V. catheter for administration. However, you may need a smaller catheter for elderly patients, those with chronic illnesses who are hospitalized frequently, or severely dehydrated patients.

Written in blood

Your facility probably has specific protocols for infusing blood and blood products. For example, a unit of whole blood — about 500 ml — or packed red blood cells (PRBCs) — about 250 ml — should infuse for no longer than 4 hours because the blood can deteriorate and become contaminated with bacteria after this time. Many facilities recommend completing a transfusion in about 2 hours. However, this rate may be too fast for pediatric and geriatric patients.

Product precautions

You'll also need to take special precautions when transfusing blood products, such as platelets, cryoprecipitate, and granulocytes. Consult your facility's procedure manual to find out the type of tubing to use and the rate and duration of the transfusion.

Cheat sheet

Blood infusions

• Filter out agglutinated cells with special administration sets.
• The drip factor is 10 to 15 gtt/ml.
• Use at least an 18G I.V. catheter.

In addition, some medical conditions require the use of special tubing. For example, cancer patients may need to use a leukocyte filter with blood products to prevent complications.

Blood cell brain teaser

Here's an example of a dosage calculation problem that involves PRBCs: Your patient is to receive 250 ml PRBCs over 4 hours. The drip factor of the tubing is 10 gtt/ml. What's the drip rate in drops per minute?

- First, find the flow rate in milliliters per minute:

$$\frac{250 \text{ ml PRBC}}{4 \text{ hours}} = \frac{62.5 \text{ ml}}{1 \text{ hour}}$$

> Use the flow rate in milliliters per hour...

$$\frac{62.5 \text{ ml}}{1 \text{ hour}} \times \frac{1 \text{ hour}}{60 \text{ minutes}} = 1.04 \text{ ml/minute} = \text{flow rate}$$

- Multiply the flow rate by the drip factor to find the drip rate in drops per minute:

$$\frac{1.04 \text{ ml}}{1 \text{ minute}} \times \frac{10 \text{ gtt}}{\text{ml}} = 10.4 \text{ gtt/minute}$$

> ...to find the drip rate in drops per minute.

The drip rate is 10.4 gtt/minute, or approximately 10 gtt/minute.

Total parenteral nutrition

A patient receives total parenteral nutrition (TPN) when his nutritional needs can't be met enterally because of elevated requirements or impaired digestion or absorption in the GI tract. TPN refers to any nutrient solution, including lipids, given through a central venous line.

TPN can be administered through a central vein, such as the subclavian vein or internal jugular vein. Peripheral parenteral nutrition, which is administered through the veins of the arms, legs, or scalp, supplies full caloric needs while avoiding the risks that accompany a central line. Most facilities have a written protocol regarding insertion sites and recommended solutions.

TPN is available as commercially prepared products or individually formulated solutions from the pharmacy. Solutions are prepared under sterile conditions to guard against patient infection. Very rarely are nurses responsible for preparing TPN solutions on the unit.

Cheat sheet

TPN administration

- Can be given centrally or peripherally
- Initially infused at 40 ml/hour then increased to maintenance
- Administer with infusion pump

Added attractions

TPN solutions contain a 10% or greater dextrose concentration. Amino acids are added to maintain or restore nitrogen balance, and vitamins, electrolytes, and trace minerals are added to meet individual patient needs.

Lipids also may be added, but they're often given separately to prevent their destruction by the other nutrients. Remember that additives increase a solution's total volume, so they affect intake measurements.

For example, when assessing the amount of fluid remaining in the TPN bottle, don't be surprised to find 20 to 50 ml more than you expected. If this happens, find out whether the volume of additives explains the discrepancy.

What goes up...must come down

Initially, TPN is infused at a slow rate — usually 40 ml/hour — which is gradually increased to a maintenance level. The rate is gradually decreased before discontinuing TPN. Most solutions are administered through an infusion pump.

For example, a patient's TPN may be increased to a maintenance level of 2,000 ml in 24 hours. To set the maintenance flow rate of the infusion pump, you need to find the hourly flow rate. To do this, simply divide the amount to be infused daily — 2,000 ml — by 24 hours. You find that you should set the infusion pump at 83 ml/hour.

Okay, enough dosage calculations. Take a rest and then give the quick quiz a go!

Quick quiz

1. To calculate the drip rate of an I.V. solution, you must first determine the:

    A.   drip factor.
    B.   flow rate.
    C.   size of the tubing.

Answer: A. The drip factor, or number of drops/milliliter of solution, depends on the administration set you're using and is listed on the set's label.

2. An I.V. of 1,000 ml is ordered to infuse over 10 hours at 25 gtt/minute. The set calibration is 15 gtt/ml. After 5 hours, 650 ml have infused instead of 500. To recalculate the flow rate for the remaining solution, you would:

    A.   slow the rate to 18 gtt/minute.
    B.   increase the rate to 35 gtt/minute.
    C.   slow the rate to 10 gtt/minute.

Answer: A. To solve this, determine the amount of fluid remaining by subtracting 650 ml from 1,000 ml. Convert the time remaining to minutes. Set up the equation using this formula:

$$\frac{\text{total ml}}{\text{total minutes}} = \text{drip factor in gtt/ml}$$

3.   The test for the therapeutic range for heparin is the:
    A.   activated partial thrombin test.
    B.   partial thromboplastin time.
    C.   partial thrombin activation test.

Answer: B. Heparin doses are individualized based on the patient's coagulation status, which is measured by this test.

4.   For a microdrip set with a drip factor of 60 gtt/ml, the drip rate is:
    A.   half the flow rate.
    B.   10 times greater than the flow rate.
    C.   the same as the flow rate.

Answer: C. The drip rate is the same as the flow rate because the number of minutes in an hour—60—is the same as the drip factor.

5.   You start a continuous infusion of 150 U of regular insulin in 150 ml of normal saline solution. If the prescribed dose is 8 U/hour, what's the flow rate?
    A.   8 ml/hour
    B.   80 ml/hour
    C.   18 ml/hour

Answer: A. Solve this problem by setting up the first fraction with the known solution strength and the second fraction with the desired dose and the unknown solution strength, putting these fractions into a proportion, cross-multiplying, and then dividing and canceling the units of measure that appear in both the numerator and denominator.

6.   The PCA pump can provide a dose of medication on demand or at a:
    A.   basil rate.
    B.   basal rate.
    C.   basic rate.

Answer: B. The basal rate is a continuous infusion administered by the PCA.

7. You need to infuse 1,500 ml of D_5W over 10 hours. What's the flow rate?

    A.   50 ml/hour

    B.   100 ml/hour

    C.   150 ml/hour

Answer: C. Set up the equation using this formula:

$$\frac{\text{total volume ordered}}{\text{number of hours}}$$

8. Your patient needs an infusion of D_5W at 75 ml/hour. If the tubing set is calibrated at 20 gtt/ml, what's the drip rate?

    A.   75 gtt/minute

    B.   25 gtt/minute

    C.   50 gtt/minute

Answer: B. Set up the equation using this formula:

$$\frac{\text{total ml}}{\text{total minutes}} \times \text{drip factor in gtt/ml}$$

Scoring

☆☆☆ If you answered all eight items correctly, excellent! Enjoy every gtt of success!

☆☆ If you answered five to seven correctly, great job! Your drip factor is beyond measure! (All right, if you insist, we'll give you 15 gtt/ml.)

☆ If you answered fewer than five correctly, no problem! Go with the flow, keep calculatin', and infuse in peace and joy!

I see three more chapters of special calculations in your future...

Part VI

Special calculations

13 Calculating pediatric dosages — 235

14 Calculating obstetric drug dosages — 255

15 Calculating critical care dosages — 269

13

Calculating pediatric dosages

Just the facts

In this chapter, you'll learn:

♦ how to prepare drugs and administer them to infants and children by the four routes

♦ how to calculate safe pediatric drug dosages according to body weight and body surface area

♦ how to apply pediatric infusion guidelines and protocols

♦ how to calculate pediatric fluid needs based on body weight, calories of metabolism, and body surface area.

A look at calculating pediatric dosages

When calculating drug dosages for pediatric patients, remember that children aren't just small adults. Because of their size, metabolism, and other factors, children have special medication needs and require special care. Also, an incorrect dose is more likely to be harmful to a child than to an adult.

Same routes, different needs

Although both children and adults receive drugs by the oral (P.O.), subcutaneous (S.C.), intramuscular (I.M.), and intravenous (I.V.) routes, the similarity ends there. The pharmacokinetics, pharmacodynamics, and pharmacotherapeutics of drugs differ greatly between children and adults.

For example, a child's immature body systems may be unable to handle certain drugs. Also, a child's total volume of body water is much greater proportionally than an adult's, so drug distribution is altered. Because of these differences, you must be especially careful when calculating special dosages for children. (See *A trio of timesaving tips*, page 236)

Why is this chapter so important? Children have special dosage calculation needs.

Administering pediatric drugs

The methods used to prepare drugs and administer them to pediatric patients also differ from the methods used for adults, depending on which route is used. There are specific administration guidelines and precautions for each route as well. (See *Giving medications to children.*)

Oral route

Infants and young children who can't swallow tablets or capsules are given oral drugs in liquid form. When a liquid preparation isn't available, generally you may crush a tablet and mix it with a small amount of liquid. Don't use essential fluids, such as infant formula, because this could lead to feeding refusal.

Remember: Never crush timed-release capsules or tablets or enteric-coated drugs. Crushing destroys the coating that causes drugs to release at the right time and prevent stomach irritation.

Measuring device advice

If a child can drink from a cup, measure and give liquid medications in a cup that's calibrated in metric and household units. If the child is very young or can't drink from a cup, use a medication dropper, syringe, or hollow-handle spoon. These devices are sold individually and also come prepackaged with some drugs.

Mix it up

If the liquid drug is prepared as a suspension or as an insoluble drug in a liquid base, mix it thoroughly before you measure and

I can't waste time

A trio of timesaving tips

When calculating safe pediatric dosages, save time and stop errors by following these suggestions:
• Carry a calculator for use when solving equations.
• Consult a formulary or drug handbook to verify a drug dose. When in doubt, call the pharmacist.
• Keep your patient's weight in kilograms at his bedside so you don't have to estimate it or weigh him in a rush.

Advice from the experts

Giving medications to children

When giving oral and parenteral medications to children, safety is essential. Keep these points in mind:
• Check the child's mouth to make sure he has swallowed the oral drug.
• Carefully mix oral drugs that come in suspension form.
• Give intramuscular (I.M.) injections in the vastus lateralis muscle of infants who haven't started walking.
• Don't inject more than 1 ml into I.M. or subcutaneous sites.
• Rotate injection sites.

Peak technique

I.M. injections for infants

When giving intramuscular (I.M.) injections to infants, use the vastus lateralis muscle. Don't inject into the gluteus muscle until it's fully developed, which occurs when the child learns to walk. These illustrations show how to give an I.M. injection using one- and two-person methods.

administer it. This ensures that none of the drug remains settled out of the solution. Whenever you give an oral drug, check the child's mouth to make sure that all of the drug was swallowed.

S.C. route

Pediatric patients also may receive childhood immunizations and drugs such as insulin by the S.C. route. When giving S.C. injections, make sure each injection contains no more than 1 ml of solution. Any area with sufficient S.C. tissue may be used—the upper arm, abdomen, and thigh are the most common.

I.M. route

Drugs for pain and sedation as well as vaccines against diphtheria, pertussis, and tetanus are commonly administered by the I.M. route. When giving I.M. injections, make sure each injection contains no more than 1 ml of solution. Give I.M. injections in the thighs of infants because their gluteal muscles don't develop until they learn to walk.

Finding the nerve

Be aware of the risk for nerve damage when selecting the site, needle length, and injection technique. (See *I.M. injections for infants*, page 237.)

I.V. route

Fluids and drugs may also be administered by the I.V. route. I.V. site placement may be in a peripheral or central vein. Because pediatric patients can tolerate only a limited amount of fluid, dilute I.V. drugs and administer I.V. fluids cautiously. Always use an infusion pump with infants and small children.

Infiltration and inflammation alert!

Inspect I.V. sites frequently for signs of infiltration (cool, blanched, and puffy skin) or inflammation (warm and reddened skin). Do this before, during, and after the infusion because children's vessels are immature and easily damaged by drugs. If infiltration occurs, stop the infusion and call the doctor.

Cheat sheet

Route guidelines

- *Oral (P.O.)*—liquid suspensions mixed first
- *Subcutaneous (S.C.)*—never more than 1 ml of solution; any area with sufficient S.C. tissue used
- *Intramuscular (I.M.)*—never more than 1 ml of solution; administered in the thigh of infants
- *I.V.*—drugs diluted carefully and administered cautiously; infusion pump used with infants and small children

Calculating dosages

To calculate and verify the safety of pediatric drug dosages, use either the dosage per kilogram of body weight method or the body surface area (BSA) method. Other methods, such as those based on age, are less accurate and typically aren't used.

Whichever method you use, remember that you're professionally and legally responsible for checking the safety of a prescribed dose prior to administration.

Dosage per kilogram of body weight

Many pharmaceutical companies provide information about safe drug dosages for pediatric patients in milligrams per kilogram of body weight. This is the most accurate and common way to calculate pediatric dosages. Pediatric dosages are usually expressed as mg/kg/day or mg/kg/dose. Based on this information, you can determine the pediatric dose by multiplying the child's weight in kilograms by the required number of milligrams of drug per kilogram.

Shifting weight: From pounds to kilograms

Because most patients' weights are measured in pounds, you must convert from pounds to kilograms before calculating the dosage per kilogram of body weight. Remember that 1 kg equals 2.2 lb.

Real world problems

The following examples show how to use proportions to convert pounds to kilograms, how to calculate mg/kg/dose for one time or as needed (p.r.n.) medications, and how to calculate mg/kg/day for doses given around-the-clock to maintain a continuous drug effect.

A weighty problem

If your 6-year-old patient weighs 41.5 lb, how much does he weigh in kilograms?

Here's how to solve this problem using ratios:

- Set up the proportion, remembering that 2.2 lb equals 1 kg:

$$X : 41.5 \text{ lb} :: 1 \text{ kg} : 2.2 \text{ lb}$$

- Multiply the extremes and the means:

$$X \times 2.2 \text{ lb} = 1 \text{ kg} \times 41.5 \text{ lb}$$

- Solve for X by dividing each side of the equation by 2.2 lb and canceling units that appear in both the numerator and denominator:

$$\frac{X \times 2.2 \, \cancel{\text{lb}}}{2.2 \, \cancel{\text{lb}}} = \frac{1 \text{ kg} \times 41.5 \, \cancel{\text{lb}}}{2.2 \, \cancel{\text{lb}}}$$

$$X = \frac{41.5 \text{ kg}}{2.2}$$

$$X = 18.9 \text{ kg}$$

The child weighs 18.9 kg, rounded off to 19 kg.

Milligram mystery

The doctor orders single dose of 20 mg/kg/dose of amoxicillin oral suspension for a toddler who weighs 20 lb (9.1 kg). What's the dose in milligrams?

Here's how to solve this problem using fractions:

- Set up the proportion with the ordered dosage in one fraction and the unknown dosage and the patient's weight in the other fraction:

$$\frac{20 \text{ mg}}{1 \text{ kg/dose}} = \frac{X}{9 \text{ kg/dose}}$$

• Cross-multiply the fractions:

$$X \times 1 \text{ kg/dose} = 20 \text{ mg} \times 9 \text{ kg/dose}$$

• Solve for X by dividing each side of the equation by 1 kg/day and canceling units that appear in both the numerator and denominator:

$$\frac{X \times 1 \, \cancel{\text{kg/dose}}}{1 \, \cancel{\text{kg/dose}}} = \frac{20 \text{ mg} \times 9 \, \cancel{\text{kg/dose}}}{1 \, \cancel{\text{kg/dose}}}$$

$$X = 180 \text{ mg}$$

The patient needs 180 mg of amoxicillin.

A perplexing penicillin problem

The doctor orders *penicillin V potassium oral suspension 56 mg/kg/day in four divided doses* for a patient who weighs 55 lb. The suspension that's available is penicillin V potassium 125 mg/5 ml. What volume should you administer for each dose?

Here's how to solve this problem using ratios and fractions:

• First, convert the child's weight from pounds to kilograms by setting up the following proportion:

$$X : 55 \text{ lb} :: 1 \text{ kg} : 2.2 \text{ lb}$$

• Multiply the extremes and the means:

$$X \times 2.2 \text{ lb} = 1 \text{ kg} \times 55 \text{ lb}$$

• Solve for X by dividing each side of the equation by 2.2 lb and canceling units that appear in both the numerator and denominator:

$$\frac{X \times 2.2 \, \cancel{\text{lb}}}{2.2 \, \cancel{\text{lb}}} = \frac{1 \text{ kg} \times 55 \, \cancel{\text{lb}}}{2.2 \, \cancel{\text{lb}}}$$

$$X = \frac{55 \text{ kg}}{2.2}$$

$$X = 25 \text{ kg}$$

• The child weighs 25 kg. Next, determine the total daily dosage by setting up a proportion with the patient's weight and the unknown dosage on one side and the ordered dosage on the other side:

$$\frac{25 \text{ kg}}{X} = \frac{1 \text{ kg}}{56 \text{ mg}}$$

• Cross-multiply the fractions:

$$X \times 1 \text{ kg} = 56 \text{ mg} \times 25 \text{ kg}$$

First, I need to figure out the child's weight in kilograms; then I can calculate the right dosage.

Next, I determine the total daily dosage.

• Solve for *X* by dividing each side of the equation by 1 kg and canceling units that appear in both the numerator and denominator:

$$\frac{X \times 1\,kg}{1\,kg} = \frac{56\,mg \times 25\,kg}{1\,kg}$$

$$X = \frac{56\,mg \times 25}{1}$$

$$X = 1,400\,mg$$

Next, I determine the dose to administer every 6 hours.

• The child's daily dosage is 1,400 mg. Now, divide the daily dosage by 4 doses to determine the dose to administer every 6 hours:

$$X = \frac{1,400\,mg}{4\,doses}$$

$$X = 350\,mg/dose$$

The child should receive 350 mg every 6 hours.

• Finally, calculate the volume to give for each dose by setting up a proportion with the unknown volume and the amount in one dose on one side and the available dose on the other side:

$$\frac{X}{350\,mg} = \frac{5\,ml}{125\,mg}$$

Finally, I determine the volume to give for each dose.

• Cross-multiply the fractions:

$$X \times 125\,mg = 5\,ml \times 350\,mg$$

• Solve for *X* by dividing each side of the equation by 125 mg and canceling units that appear in both the numerator and denominator:

$$\frac{X \times 125\,mg}{125\,mg} = \frac{5\,ml \times 350\,mg}{125\,mg}$$

$$X = \frac{5\,ml \times 350}{125}$$

$$X = \frac{1,750\,ml}{125}$$

$$X = 14\,ml$$

You should administer 14 ml of the drug at each dose.

Yeah! Right on the dose...er, nose!

Dosage by BSA

The BSA method is used to calculate safe pediatric dosages for a limited number of drugs. (It's also used to calculate safe dosages for adult patients receiving extremely potent drugs or drugs requiring great precision, such as antineoplastic or chemotherapeutic agents.)

BSA plot thickens

Calculating dosages by BSA involves two steps:

☞ Plot the patient's height and weight on a chart called a *nomogram*, to determine the BSA in square meters (m^2). (See *What's in a nomogram?*)

✌ Multiply the BSA by the prescribed pediatric dose in $mg/m^2/day$.

Here's the formula:

$$\text{child's dose in mg} = \text{child's BSA in } m^2 \times \frac{\text{pediatric dose in mg}}{m^2/day}$$

The BSA method can also be used to calculate a child's dose based on the average adult BSA — 1.73 m^2 — and an average adult dose.

The formula looks like this:

$$\text{child's dose in mg} = \frac{\text{child's BSA in } m^2}{\text{average adult BSA (1.73 } m^2)} \times \text{average adult dose}$$

Real world problems

The following problems show how these two formulas are used in the BSA method of dosage calculation.

An engrossing ephedrine equation

The doctor orders *100 mg/m^2/day of ephedrine* for a child who is 40″ tall and weighs 64 lb. How much ephedrine should the child receive daily?

• Use the nomogram to determine that the child's BSA is 0.96 m^2.

• Using the appropriate formula above, determine the daily dosage:

$$X = 0.96 \, m^2 \times \frac{100 \text{ mg}}{1 \, m^2/day}$$

Cheat sheet

BSA

• Measured in m^2
• Determined through intersection of height and weight on nomogram
• Multiply by the prescribed dose in $mg/m^2/day$ to calculate safe pediatric dosages

The Real World

> *Peak technique*

What's in a nomogram?

Body surface area (BSA) is critical when calculating dosages for pediatric patients or for drugs that are extremely potent and need to be given in precise amounts. The nomogram shown here lets you plot the patient's height and weight to determine the BSA. Here's how it works:

• Locate the patient's height in the left column of the nomogram and his weight in the right column.

• Use a ruler to draw a straight line connecting the two points. The point where the line intersects the surface area column indicates the patient's BSA in square meters.

• For an average-sized child, use the simplified nomogram in the box. Just find the child's weight in pounds on the left side of the scale, and then read the corresponding BSA on the right side.

- Solve for X:

$$X = 0.96 \text{ m}^2 \times \frac{100 \text{ mg}}{1 \text{ m}^2/\text{day}}$$

$$X = 96 \text{ mg/day}$$

The child needs 96 mg of ephedrine per day.

A captivating chemotherapy question

A child who needs chemotherapy is 36″ tall and weighs 40 lb. What's the safe drug dose if the average adult dose is 1,000 mg?
- Use the nomogram to determine that the child's BSA is 0.72 m².
- Then set up an equation using the appropriate formula from above. Divide the child's BSA by 1.73 m² (the average adult BSA), and multiply by the average adult dose, 1,000 mg:

$$X = \frac{0.72 \text{ m}^2}{1.73 \text{ m}^2} \times 1,000 \text{ mg}$$

- Solve for X by canceling units that appear in both the numerator and denominator, multiplying the child's BSA by the average adult dose, and dividing the result by the average adult BSA:

$$X = \frac{0.72 \text{ m}^2 \times 1,000 \text{ mg}}{1.73 \text{ m}^2}$$

$$X = 416 \text{ mg}$$

The safe dose for this child is 416 mg.

Verifying calculations

Although the doctor determines the medication dosage, the nurse, as an important "last line of defense," verifies that the ordered dosage is safe. Some nursing drug handbooks contain usual (recommended) pediatric dosages for commonly prescribed drugs. The pharmacist is another excellent resource for verifying drug safety.

Real world problems

Here's a real world example of verifying calculations: The doctor orders *chloral hydrate 75 mg P.O.* to sedate a 3 kg neonate for an electroencephalogram. The drug resource states the usual (recommended) dosage of chloral hydrate for a neonate is 25 mg/kg/dose

the Real World

for sedation prior to a procedure. Here's how to solve this problem using fractions:
• Set up the proportion with the usual dosage in one fraction and the unknown dosage and the patient's weight in the other fraction:

$$\frac{25 \text{ mg}}{1 \text{ kg/dose}} = \frac{X}{3 \text{ kg/dose}}$$

• Cross-multiply the fractions:

$$X \times 1 \text{ kg/dose} = 25 \text{ mg} \times 3 \text{ kg/dose}$$

• Solve for X by dividing each side of the equation by 1 kg/dose and canceling units that appear in both the numerator and denominator:

$$\frac{X \times 1 \text{ kg/dose}}{1 \text{ kg/dose}} = \frac{25 \text{ mg} \times 3 \text{ kg/dose}}{1 \text{ kg/dose}}$$

$$X = 75 \text{ mg}$$

The patient needs 75 mg of chloral hydrate. That's what the doctor ordered and, therefore, the dose is safe to administer.

Penicillin puzzler

The doctor orders *penicillin V potassium oral suspension 250 mg P.O. q 6 hr* for a patient who weighs 55 lb. Is the dose safe? The suspension that's available is penicillin V potassium 125 mg/5 ml. What volume should you administer for each dose?

Here's how to answer these questions using ratios and fractions:
• First, convert the child's weight from pounds to kilograms by setting up the following proportion:

$$X : 55 \text{ lb} :: 1 \text{ kg} : 2.2 \text{ lb}$$

• Multiply the extremes and the means:

$$X \times 2.2 \text{ lb} = 1 \text{ kg} \times 55 \text{ lb}$$

• Solve for X by dividing each side of the equation by 2.2 lb and canceling units that appear in both the numerator and denominator:

$$\frac{X \times 2.2 \text{ lb}}{2.2 \text{ lb}} = \frac{1 \text{ kg} \times 55 \text{ lb}}{2.2 \text{ lb}}$$

$$X = \frac{55 \text{ kg}}{2.2}$$

$$X = 25 \text{ kg}$$

The child weighs 25 kg.

- Now verify the usual (recommended) dosage. The drug reference states to give penicillin V potassium 25 to 50 mg/kg/day orally in divided doses every 6 to 8 hours. This indicates a safe daily dosage range — a low dosage (25 mg/kg/day) and a high dosage (50 mg/kg/day). These are also the minimum (low dosage) and the maximum (high dosage) dosages for the day.

- Next, determine the usual total daily dosage range by setting up two proportions with the patient's weight on one side and the usual dosage (either the low dosage and or the high dosage) on the other side. Let's look at the high dose first:

$$\frac{25 \text{ kg}}{X} = \frac{1 \text{ kg}}{50 \text{ mg}}$$

- Cross-multiply the fractions:

$$X \times 1 \text{ kg} = 50 \text{ mg} \times 25 \text{ kg}$$

- Solve for X by dividing each side of the equation by 1 kg and canceling units that appear in both the numerator and denominator:

$$\frac{X \times \cancel{1 \text{ kg}}}{\cancel{1 \text{ kg}}} = \frac{50 \text{ mg} \times 25 \cancel{\text{ kg}}}{1 \cancel{\text{ kg}}}$$

$$X = \frac{50 \text{ mg} \times 25}{1}$$

$$X = 1{,}250 \text{ mg}$$

- The child's maximum daily dosage is 1,250 mg. Now divide the daily dosage by four doses to determine the maximum safe dose to administer every 6 hours:

$$X = \frac{1{,}250 \text{ mg}}{4 \text{ doses}}$$

$$X = 312.5 \text{ mg/dose or } 313 \text{ mg/dose}$$

- Now repeat the same steps to determine the low or minimum dose:

$$\frac{25 \text{ kg}}{X} = \frac{1 \text{ kg}}{25 \text{ mg}}$$

- Cross-multiply the fractions:

$$X \times 1 \text{ kg} = 25 \text{ mg} \times 25 \text{ kg}$$

- Solve for X by dividing each side of the equation by 1 kg and canceling like units:

$$\frac{X \times 1\text{kg}}{1\text{kg}} = \frac{25\text{ mg} \times 25\text{ kg}}{1\text{ kg}}$$

$$X = \frac{25\text{ mg} \times 25}{1}$$

$$X = 625\text{ mg}$$

• The child's minimum daily dosage is 625 mg. Now divide the daily dosage by four doses to determine the minimum safe dose to administer every 6 hours:

$$X = \frac{625\text{ mg}}{4\text{ doses}}$$

$$X = 156.25 \text{ or } 156\text{ mg/dose}$$

The safe daily dosage range is 625 mg to 1,250 mg for this child. The doctor ordered 250 mg every 6 hours (or four doses per day) or a total dosage of 1,000 mg (250 mg/dose × four doses). This falls within the safe daily range.

• The child can safely receive 250 mg every 6 hours. Finally, calculate the volume to give for each dose by setting up a proportion with the unknown volume and the amount in one dose on one side and the available dose on the other side:

$$\frac{X}{250\text{ mg}} = \frac{5\text{ ml}}{125\text{ mg}}$$

$$X \times 125\text{ mg} = 5\text{ ml} \times 250\text{ mg}$$

YES!

• Solve for X by dividing each side of the equation by 125 mg and canceling units that appear in both the numerator and denominator:

$$\frac{X \times 125\text{ mg}}{125\text{ mg}} = \frac{5\text{ ml} \times 250\text{ mg}}{125\text{ mg}}$$

$$X = \frac{5\text{ ml} \times 250}{125}$$

$$X = \frac{1,250\text{ ml}}{125}$$

$$X = 10\text{ ml}$$

You should administer 10 ml of the drug at each dose.

I.V. guidelines

Because pediatric I.V. drug administration is so complex, be sure to follow all written guidelines and protocols about dosages, fluid volumes for dilution, and administration rates.

I.V. fluids and drugs are administered by continuous or intermittent infusion.

Continuous infusions

A continuous infusion is used when the pediatric patient requires around-the-clock fluids, drug therapy, or both. Fluids may be infused to maintain volume or to correct an existing fluid or electrolyte imbalance.

To prepare for a continuous drug infusion, add the drug to a small-volume bag of I.V. fluid — be sure to carefully follow the manufacturer's guidelines for mixing the solution. Remember that pediatric patients can tolerate only small amounts of fluid.

Five fundamental steps

Follow these steps to start a continuous infusion:

☝ Calculate the dosage.

✌ Draw up the drug in a syringe; then add the drug to the I.V. bag through the drug additive port, using aseptic technique.

🖐 Mix the drug thoroughly.

🖐 Label the I.V. bag with the drug's name, the dosage, the time and date it was mixed, and your initials.

🖐 Hang the solution and administer the drug by infusion pump at the prescribed flow rate.

Intermittent infusions

Intermittent infusion is used frequently today in both acute care and home care settings. If the pediatric patient is capable of normal enteral fluid intake, I.V. fluids or drug infusions may only be necessary at periodic intervals. A vascular access device can be kept in place, eliminating the need for continuous fluid infusion. The child can remain mobile, minimizing the potential for volume overload.

Usually, a volume-control device such as the Buretrol set, which maintains flow rate by using a positive-pressure pumping

Intermittent I.V. infusion control

Accurate fluid administration is extremely important for pediatric patients. So syringes, infusion pumps, and other volume-control devices are used extensively to regulate intermittent I.V. infusions. One typical device, the Buretrol set, is shown below.

mechanism, is used for intermittent infusion. A small-volume bag of I.V. fluid with a microdrip set is another option. (See *Intermittent I.V. infusion control.*)

Adjusting the volume

Volume-control devices have 100- to 150-ml fluid chambers, which are calibrated in 1-ml increments to allow accurate fluid administration. Medication-filled syringes with microtubing can also be used to infuse small volumes via syringe pumps. Accuracy is especially important with pediatric patients because children can't tolerate as much fluid as adults and are more prone to fluid and electrolyte imbalances. The rate of I.V. infusion must be carefully controlled to ensure proper absorption and to prevent or minimize toxicity associated with rapid infusion.

Nine notable steps

If you're using a volume-control device, follow these steps to start an intermittent infusion:
• Carefully calculate the prescribed volume of drug. Some facilities consider the drug volume as part of the diluent volume. For example, if 100 mg of a drug is contained in 5 ml of fluid and the total fluid volume should be 50 ml, add 45 ml of diluent because 45 ml of diluent plus 5 ml of fluid drug volume equals a total of 50 ml.
• After careful calculation, draw up the prescribed volume of drug into a syringe.
• Add the drug to the fluid chamber through the drug additive port, using aseptic technique.
• Mix the drug thoroughly.
• Attach the volume-control device to an electronic infusion pump to control the infusion rate. If you're using a small-volume I.V. bag instead of a volume-control device and pump, use a microdrip set, which has a drip factor of 60 gtt/ml.
• Calculate the appropriate flow rate and infuse the drug.
• Label the volume-control device with the name of the drug.
• When the infusion is complete, flush the line to clear the tubing of the drug. A specific flush volume may either be ordered by the doctor or a standard volume protocol is followed based on the tubing volume, the patient's condition, or both. Administer the flush at the same rate as the drug. Label the volume-control device to indicate that the flush is infusing.
• With an intermittent infusion, disconnect the device when the flush is complete.
• During the infusion, check the I.V. site frequently for infiltration because children's veins are more prone to this problem.

Calculating pediatric fluid needs

Children's fluid needs are proportionally greater than those of adults, so children are more vulnerable to changes in fluid and electrolyte balance. Because their extracellular fluid has a higher percentage of water, children's fluid exchange rates are two to three times greater than those of adults, leaving them more susceptible to dehydration.

Three ways to figure fluids

Determining and meeting the fluid needs of children are important nursing responsibilities. You can calculate the number of milliliters of fluid a child needs based on:
- weight in kilograms
- metabolism (calories required)
- BSA in square meters.

Although results may vary slightly, all three methods are appropriate. Keep in mind that fluid replacement also can be affected by clinical conditions that cause fluid retention or loss. Children with these conditions should receive fluids based on their individual needs.

Wow! A child's fluid exchange rate is two to three times greater than an adult's.

Fluid needs based on weight

You may use three different formulas to calculate a child's fluid needs based on his weight.

Fluid formula for tiny tots

A child who weighs less than 10 kg requires 100 ml of fluid per kilogram of body weight. To determine this child's fluid needs, first convert his weight from pounds to kilograms. Then multiply the results by 100 ml/kg/day.

Here's the formula:

$$\text{weight in kg} \times 100\ \text{ml/kg/day} = \text{fluid needs in ml/day}$$

Fluid formula for middleweights

A child weighing 10 to 20 kg requires 1,000 ml of fluid per day for the first 10 kg plus 50 ml for every kilogram over 10. To determine this child's fluid needs, follow these steps:
- Convert his weight from pounds to kilograms.
- Subtract 10 kg from the child's total weight, and then multiply the result by 50 ml/kg/day to find the child's additional fluid needs.

Here's the formula:

(total kg − 10 kg) × 50 ml/kg/day = additional fluid need in ml/day

• Add the additional daily fluid need to the 1,000 ml/day required for the first 10 kg. The total is the child's daily fluid requirement:

1,000 ml/day + additional fluid need = fluid needs in ml/day

Fluid formula for bigger kids

A child weighing more than 20 kg requires 1,500 ml of fluid for the first 20 kg plus 20 ml for each additional kilogram. To determine this child's fluid needs, follow these steps:
• Convert the child's weight from pounds to kilograms.
• Subtract 20 kg from the child's total weight, and then multiply the result by 20 ml/kg to find the child's additional fluid needs.
    Here's the formula:

(total kg − 20 kg) × 20 ml/kg/day = additional fluid need in ml/day

• Because the child needs 1,500 ml of fluid per day for the first 20 kg, add the additional fluid need to 1,500 ml. The total is the child's daily fluid requirement:

1,500 ml/day + additional fluid need = fluid needs in ml/day

Use the information above to solve the following problem.

Finding a fluid solution

How much fluid should you give a 44-lb patient over 24 hours to meet his maintenance needs?
• First, convert 44 lb to kilograms by setting up a proportion with fractions. (Remember that 1 kg equals 2.2 lb.)

$$\frac{44 \text{ lb}}{X} = \frac{2.2 \text{ lb}}{1 \text{ kg}}$$

• Cross-multiply the fractions, and then solve for X by dividing both sides of the equation by 2.2 lb and canceling units that appear in both the numerator and denominator:

$$X \times 2.2 \text{ lb} = 44 \text{ lb} \times 1 \text{ kg}$$

$$\frac{X \times 2.2 \text{ lb}}{2.2 \text{ lb}} = \frac{44 \text{ lb} \times 1 \text{ kg}}{2.2 \text{ lb}}$$

Weight-based formulas for fluid needs

• A child weighing less than 10 kg: weight in kg × 100 ml = fluid needs in ml/day
• A child weighing 10 to 20 kg: (total kg − 10 kg) × 50 ml = additional fluid need in ml/day; 1,000 ml/day + additional fluid need = fluid needs in ml/day
• A child weighing more that 20 kg: (total kg − 20 kg) × 20 ml = additional fluid need in ml/day; 1,500 ml/day + additional fluid need = fluid needs in ml/day

$$X = \frac{44 \text{ kg}}{2.2}$$

$$X = 20 \text{ kg}$$

• The child weighs 20 kg. Now, subtract 10 kg from the child's weight, and multiply the result by 50 ml/kg/day to find the child's additional fluid needs:

$$X = (20 \text{ kg} - 10 \text{ kg}) \times 50 \text{ ml/kg/day}$$

$$X = 10 \text{ kg} \times 50 \text{ ml/kg/day}$$

$$X = 500 \text{ ml/day additional fluid need}$$

• Next, add the additional fluid need to the 1,000 ml/day required for the first 10 kg (because the child weighs between 10 and 20 kg).

$$X = 1{,}000 \text{ ml/day} + 500 \text{ ml/day}$$

$$X = 1{,}500 \text{ ml/day}$$

The child should receive 1,500 ml of fluid in 24 hours to meet his fluid maintenance needs.

Look closely! I can cancel kg in this equation to find the child's additional fluid need in ml/day.

Fluid needs based on calories

You can calculate fluid needs based on calories because water is necessary for metabolism. A child should receive 120 ml of fluid for every 100 kilocalories (kcal) of metabolism, also commonly called calories.

Fluids help burn calories

To calculate fluid requirements based on calorie requirements, follow these steps:
• Find the child's calorie requirements. You can take this from a table of recommended dietary allowances for children, or you can have a dietitian calculate it.
• Divide the calorie requirements by 100 kcal because fluid requirements are determined for every 100 calories.
• Multiply the results by 120 ml — the amount of fluid required for every 100 kcal. Here's the formula:

$$\text{fluid requirements in ml/day} = \frac{\text{calorie requirements}}{100 \text{ kcal}} \times 120 \text{ ml}$$

Use the information above to solve the following problem.

Cheat sheet

Calorie-based formula for fluid needs

• Fluid to calorie ratio: 120 ml per 100 kcal
• Fluid requirements in ml/day = (calorie requirements ÷ 100 kcal) × 120 ml

Calorie-conscious problem

Your pediatric patient uses 900 calories/day. What are his daily fluid requirements?
• Set up the formula inserting the appropriate numbers and substituting X for the unknown amount of fluid:

$$X = \frac{900 \ \cancel{kcal}}{100 \ \cancel{kcal}} \times 120 \ ml$$

$$X = 9 \times 120 \ ml$$

$$X = 1,080 \ ml$$

The patient needs 1,080 ml of fluid per day.

Cheat sheet

BSA-based formula for fluid needs

• *For a nondehydrated child:* fluid maintenance needs in ml/day = BSA in m^2 $\times$ 1,500 ml/day/m^2

Fluid needs based on BSA

Another method for determining pediatric maintenance fluid requirements is based on the child's BSA. To calculate the daily fluid needs of a child who isn't dehydrated, multiply the BSA by 1,500, as shown in this formula:

fluid maintenance needs in ml/day = BSA in m^2 $\times$ 1,500 ml/day/m^2

Use this formula to solve the following problem.

BSA-based problem

Your patient is 36″ tall and weighs 40 lb. If his BSA is 0.72 m^2, how much fluid does he need each day?
• Set up the equation, inserting the appropriate numbers and substituting X for the unknown amount of fluid. Then solve for X:

$$X = 0.72 \ \cancel{m^2} \times 1,500 \ ml/day/\cancel{m^2}$$

$$X = 1,080 \ ml/day$$

The child needs 1,080 ml of fluid per day.

Quick quiz

1. If the suggested pediatric dosage for a drug is 35 mg/kg/day, the amount to give an infant weighing 5 kg is:
    A.   250 mg.
    B.   175 mg.
    C.   75 mg.

Answer: B. To solve this problem, set up a proportion with the suggested dosage in one ratio and the unknown quantity in the other. Multiply the means and extremes and then divide each side of the equation by the value that appears on the X side of the equation. Cancel units that appear in the numerator and denominator.

2. A child who uses 1,000 calories per day has daily fluid requirements of:
    A.   1,000 ml.
    B.   200 ml.
    C.   1,200 ml.

Answer: C. Use the equation for calculating fluid needs based on kilocalories, inserting the appropriate numbers. Then solve for X.

3. If a patient is 40″ tall, weighs 64 lb, and has a BSA of 0.96 m², how much fluid does he require per day?
    A.   1,400 ml
    B.   140 ml
    C.   1,440 ml

Answer: C. Use the equation for calculating fluid needs based on BSA, inserting the appropriate numbers. Then solve for X.

4. Your patient weighs 8 kg. What are his daily fluid needs?
    A.   1,000 ml/day
    B.   700 ml/day
    C.   800 ml/day

Answer: C. Set up the equation using the formula weight in kilograms multiplied by 100 ml/kg/day. Cancel like units.

$$8 \text{ kg} \times 100 \text{ ml/kg/day}$$

$$800 \text{ ml/day}$$

5. The chart used to determine BSA is the:
    A.   monogram.
    B.   nomogram.
    C.   pediagram.

Answer: B. A nomogram lets you plot the patient's height and weight to determine the BSA.

Scoring

☆☆☆ If you answered all five items correctly, way to go! You're the pride and joy of precise pediatric dosages!

☆☆ If you answered three to four correctly, we're impressed! There's nothing infantile about your abilities!

☆ If you answered fewer than three correctly, review and try again. You'll be a specialist in special calculations before you know it!

Calculating obstetric drug dosages

Just the facts

In this chapter, you'll learn:

♦ how to assess the mother and fetus during medication administration

♦ common obstetric drugs and their adverse effects

♦ how to calculate obstetric dosages.

A look at obstetric drug administration

During pregnancy, labor and delivery, and postpartum, drugs are commonly given to the mother for four reasons:

  to control pregnancy-induced hypertension

  to inhibit preterm labor

  to induce labor

  to prevent postpartum hemorrhage.

Because drugs administered to the mother before delivery can also affect the fetus, both mother and fetus require meticulous monitoring. *Remember:* You're caring for two patients at once, so there's a narrow margin for error.

Assessing the mother and fetus

When administering medications, frequently check the mother's vital signs, urine output, uterine contractions, and deep tendon reflexes. Carefully assess fluid intake and output along with breath sounds to reduce the mother's risk for fluid overload, which can lead to acute pulmonary edema. (See *Assessing the mother's body systems*, page 256.)

Peak technique

Assessing the mother's body systems

Assessment is a critical part of obstetric nursing. Here's what to assess in each of the mother's body systems.

Neurologic system
- Deep tendon reflexes when magnesium sulfate is infusing
- Pain
- Orientation — disorientation can indicate hypoxemia or water intoxication

Cardiovascular system
- Vital signs
- Extremities for peripheral edema with large-volume infusions
- Pulses and skin temperature in the lower extremities for evidence of deep vein thrombosis; also for Homans' sign by dorsiflexing the foot while supporting the leg — deep calf pain indicates thrombophlebitis
- I.V. site to prevent infiltration

Respiratory system
- Breath sounds
- Need for oxygen
- Lungs for pulmonary edema with large-volume infusions

GI system
- Abdomen for contractions when oxytocin is infusing
- Abdomen for bowel sounds after delivery
- Ability to pass flatus or move bowels before discharge

Genitourinary system
- Urine output
- Fluid balance to check for decreased renal function

Fluid monitoring is especially critical in women with pregnancy-induced hypertension, which can cause decreased renal function. It's also important with drugs given to inhibit preterm labor due to their antidiuretic effect.

The fetus is also the focus

While you're evaluating the mother, be sure to evaluate the fetus's response to drug therapy. Constantly assess fetal heart tones and heart rate by connecting the mother to an electronic fetal monitor. This monitor records the heart rate and also provides a tracing of it.

Be alert for a sudden increase or decrease in fetal heart rate, which may signal an adverse reaction to treatment. If either of these occur, discontinue the drug immediately. (See *It's got a good beat: Contractions and fetal heart rate.*)

Common obstetric drugs

Drugs used during pregnancy, labor and delivery, and the postpartum period include:
- terbutaline (Brethine)
- magnesium sulfate
- oxytocin (Pitocin).

Cheat sheet

Fetal heart rate

- Monitor during mother's drug therapy.
- If *sudden increase or decrease* occurs, immediately discontinue the drug.

Advice from the experts

It's got a good beat: Contractions and fetal heart rate

While you're monitoring the mother's contractions, assess the fetal heart rate, too. Follow these steps.

1. Evaluate the mother's contraction pattern.

2. Note the characteristics of the contractions.
• What's the frequency?
• What's the duration?
• What's the intensity?

3. Evaluate the fetal heart rate after establishing a baseline.
• Is the rate within normal range?
• Is tachycardia present?
• Is bradycardia present?

4. Determine the fetal heart rate variability.
• What's the short-term variability?
• What's the long-term variability?

5. Assess for changes in fetal heart rate characteristics.
• Is acceleration or increased heart rate present with contractions?
• Is deceleration or decreased heart rate present with contractions?
• Is the heart rate waveform regular and uniform in shape?
• Is the heart rate waveform irregular in shape?

Terbutaline

Terbutaline is used to inhibit preterm labor. It stimulates the beta$_2$-adrenergic receptors in the uterine smooth muscle and inhibits contractility.

Preventing preterm limits

To administer this drug, mix it in a compatible I.V. solution and administer it through an infusion pump. Then titrate the dose every 10 minutes until the contractions subside, the maximum dose is reached, or the patient is unable to tolerate the drug due to its adverse effects.

Magnesium sulfate

Another drug used during labor and delivery is magnesium sulfate, which prevents or controls seizures that may be caused by pregnancy-induced hypertension. The drug may decrease acetylcholine levels, but its exact anticonvulsant mechanism is unknown.

Controlling seizures

To administer magnesium sulfate, first give a loading dose (a high dose given over a short time to rapidly reach a therapeutic drug level). This should be followed by an infusion at a lower dose, as prescribed.

(Text continues on page 260.)

Before you give that drug!

The lowdown on three obstetric drugs

This table lists some common drugs used in the obstetric setting along with their actions, adverse reactions, and nursing considerations.

Drug	Action	Adverse reactions	Nursing considerations
oxytocin (Pitocin)	Causes potent and selective stimulation of uterine and mammary gland smooth muscle	**Maternal** • *Blood:* afibrinogenemia (may be related to postpartum bleeding) • *Central nervous system (CNS):* subarachnoid hemorrhage resulting from hypertension; seizures or coma resulting from water intoxication • *Cardiovascular (CV):* hypotension, increased heart rate, systemic venous return, increased cardiac output, arrhythmias • *Other:* hypersensitivity, tetanic uterine contractions, abruptio placentae, impaired uterine blood flow, increased uterine motility, uterine rupture **Fetal** • *Blood:* hyperbilirubinemia, hypercapnia • *CV:* bradycardia, tachycardia, premature ventricular contractions, variable deceleration of heart rate • *Other:* hypoxia, asphyxia, death • *CNS:* brain damage, seizures • *EENT:* retinal hemorrhage • *GI:* hepatic necrosis	• Oxytocin is contraindicated in cephalopelvic disproportion; where delivery requires conversion, as in transverse lie; in fetal distress; when delivery isn't imminent; and in other obstetric emergencies. • Administer by piggyback infusion so drug can be discontinued without interrupting I.V. line. *Don't give by I.V. bolus injection.* • Don't infuse in more than one site. • Monitor and record uterine contractions, heart rate, blood pressure, intrauterine pressure, fetal heart rate, and character of blood loss every 15 minutes. • Have magnesium sulfate (20% solution) available for relaxation of myometrium. • Monitor fluid intake and output. Antidiuretic effect may lead to fluid overload, seizures, and coma.

The lowdown on three obstetric drugs (continued)

Drug	Action	Adverse reactions	Nursing considerations
terbutaline (Brethine)	Relaxes uterine muscle by acting on beta₂-adrenergic receptors; inhibits uterine contractions	**Maternal** • *Blood:* increased liver enzymes • *CNS:* seizures, nervousness, tremor, headache, drowsiness, flushing, sweating • *CV:* increased heart rate, changes in blood pressure, palpitations, chest discomfort • *EENT:* tinnitus • *GI:* nausea, vomiting, altered taste • *Respiratory:* dyspnea, wheezing	• Use cautiously in patients with diabetes, hypertension, hyperthyroidism, severe cardiac disease, and arrhythmias. • Protect from light. *Don't use if discolored.* • Explain the need for the drug to the patient and family. • Give S.C. injection in lateral deltoid area. • Warn the patient about the possibility of paradoxical bronchospasm. • Tell the patient she may use tablets and aerosol concomitantly. • Tell the patient how to administer a metered dose. • Although not approved by the Food and Drug Administration for treatment of preterm labor, this drug is considered very effective and is used in many hospitals. • Monitor the neonate for hypoglycemia. • Monitor the patient's blood glucose level with long-term use.
magnesium sulfate	May decrease acetylcholine released by nerve impulse, but anticonvulsant mechanisms unknown	**Maternal** • *CNS:* sweating, drowsiness, depressed reflexes, flaccid paralysis, hypothermia, flushing • *CV:* hypotension, circulatory collapse, depressed cardiac function, heart block • *Other:* fatal respiratory paralysis, hypocalcemia with tetany	• Use cautiously during labor and in patients with impaired renal function, myocardial damage, or heart block. • This drug can decrease the frequency and force of uterine contractions. • Keep calcium gluconate available to reverse magnesium sulfate intoxication. • Use cautiously in patients undergoing digitalization because arrhythmias may occur. • Watch for respiratory depression. • Monitor intake and output. • Monitor deep tendon reflexes. • Monitor the neonate for magnesium sufate toxicity. • Maximum infusion is 150 mg/minute. • Signs of hypermagnesemia begin to appear at blood levels of 4 mEq/L. • This drug may be used as a tocolytic agent to inhibit premature labor. • This drug should be stopped at least 2 hours before delivery to avoid fetal respiratory depression.

During the infusion, closely assess knee jerk and patellar reflexes; loss of these signals drug toxicity. If toxicity occurs, the doctor will probably order calcium gluconate as an antidote.

Oxytocin

Oxytocin — the drug most commonly used to induce labor — selectively stimulates uterine smooth muscle.

Compelling contractions

After mixing oxytocin with a compatible solution, administer it by I.V. infusion pump and titrate until a normal contraction pattern occurs. When labor is firmly established, the doctor may prescribe a decrease in the infusion rate. Carefully monitor contraction strength because the drug can cause severe contractions that can lead to uterine rupture as well as fetal and maternal death.

Blocking bleeding

Oxytocin also may be used to control bleeding after delivery of the placenta. To accomplish this, add the drug to 1 L of I.V. fluid, and then infuse it at a rate that controls bleeding but doesn't exceed 20 milliunits (mU) per minute. (See *The lowdown on three obstetric drugs*, pages 258 and 259.)

Dosage calculations

In the labor and delivery unit, you must be especially careful to calculate and administer drugs accurately. For one thing, you may be dealing with life-threatening problems, such as hemorrhage and seizures caused by pregnancy-induced hypertension.

Administering accurate dosages to the mother helps avoid fetal complications. Be sure to examine drug labels closely. They contain valuable information for calculating dosages. (See *Learn from labels*.)

Real world problems

The examples below show how to calculate obstetric drugs using proportions.

Overdue? Order oxytocin.

Your patient is 10 days overdue, so the doctor prescribes oxytocin to stimulate labor. The order reads *1 ml (10 U) oxytocin in 1 L (1,000 ml) NSS; infuse via pump at 2 mU/minute for 20 minutes, then increase flow rate to 3 mU/minute.* What's the solu-

the Real World

tion's concentration? What's the flow rate needed to deliver
2 mU/minute for 20 minutes? What's the flow rate needed to deliver 3 mU/minute thereafter?

• Determine the concentration of the solution by setting up a proportion with the ordered concentration in one fraction and the unknown concentration in the other fraction:

$$\frac{10 \text{ U}}{1,000 \text{ ml}} = \frac{X}{1 \text{ ml}}$$

• Cross-multiply the fractions:

$$X \times 1,000 \text{ ml} = 10 \text{ U} \times 1 \text{ ml}$$

• Solve for X by dividing both sides of the equation by 1,000 ml and canceling units that appear in both the numerator and denominator:

$$\frac{X \times 1,000 \text{ ml}}{1,000 \text{ ml}} = \frac{10 \text{ U} \times 1 \text{ ml}}{1,000 \text{ ml}}$$

$$X = \frac{10 \text{ U}}{1,000}$$

$$X = 0.01 \text{ U}$$

• The amount 0.01 U can be written in milliunits (mU): 1 mU is 1/1,000 of a unit; 1,000 mU is 1 U. Therefore, 0.01 U times 1,000 equals 10 mU. So, the concentration is 10 mU/ml.

First, I determine the concentration of the solution.

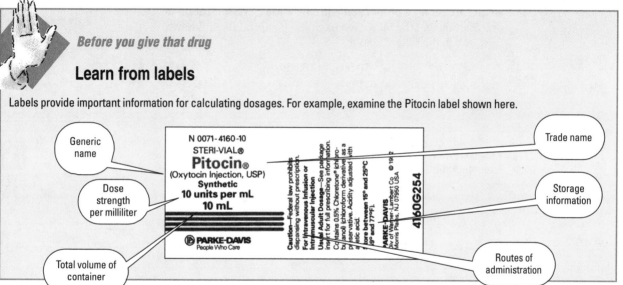

Before you give that drug

Learn from labels

Labels provide important information for calculating dosages. For example, examine the Pitocin label shown here.

Generic name

Dose strength per milliliter

Total volume of container

Trade name

Storage information

Routes of administration

N 0071-4160-10
STERI-VIAL®
Pitocin®
(Oxytocin Injection, USP)
Synthetic
10 units per mL
10 mL

Ⓟ **PARKE-DAVIS**
People Who Care

Caution—Federal law prohibits dispensing without prescription.
See package insert for full prescribing information.
For Intravenous Infusion or Intramuscular Injection
Usual Adult Dosage—See package insert for full prescribing information.
Contains 0.5% Chlorobutanol (chloro-butanol) chloroform derivative as a preservative. Acidity adjusted with acetic acid.
Store between 15° and 25°C (59° and 77°F).

PARKE-DAVIS
Div of Warner-Lambert Co.
Morris Plains, NJ 07950 USA

4160G254

- Next, determine the flow rate. If the prescribed dosage of oxytocin is 2 mU/minute for 20 minutes, the patient receives a total of 40 mU. To calculate the rate needed to provide that dose, set up a proportion with the known concentration in one fraction and the total oxytocin dose and unknown flow rate in the other:

$$\frac{10 \text{ mU}}{1 \text{ ml}} = \frac{40 \text{ mU}}{X}$$

- Cross-multiply the fractions:

$$X \times 10 \text{ mU} = 1 \text{ ml} \times 40 \text{ mU}$$

- Solve for X by dividing both sides of the equation by 10 mU and canceling units that appear in both the numerator and denominator:

$$\frac{X \times \cancel{10 \text{ mU}}}{\cancel{10 \text{ mU}}} = \frac{1 \text{ ml} \times 40 \cancel{\text{ mU}}}{10 \cancel{\text{ mU}}}$$

$$X = \frac{40 \text{ ml}}{10}$$

$$X = 4 \text{ ml}$$

- The flow rate is 4 ml/20 minutes. Because this drug must be delivered by infusion pump, compute the hourly flow rate by multiplying the 20-minute rate by 3:

$$4 \text{ ml/20 minutes} \times 3 = 12 \text{ ml/hour}$$

- The hourly flow rate is 12 ml/hour. Finally, calculate the flow rate to be used after the first 20 minutes, resulting in 3 mU/minute (180 mU/hour). Having calculated the solution's concentration as 10 mU/ml, set up a proportion with the known concentration in one fraction and the increased oxytocin dose and the unknown flow rate in the other fraction:

$$\frac{10 \text{ mU}}{1 \text{ ml}} = \frac{180 \text{ mU}}{X}$$

- Cross-multiply the fractions:

$$X \times 10 \text{ mU} = 1 \text{ ml} \times 180 \text{ mU}$$

- Solve for X by dividing both sides of the equation by 10 mU and canceling units that appear in both the numerator and denominator:

$$\frac{X \times \cancel{10 \text{ mU}}}{\cancel{10 \text{ mU}}} = \frac{1 \text{ ml} \times 180 \cancel{\text{ mU}}}{10 \cancel{\text{ mU}}}$$

$$X = \frac{180 \text{ ml}}{10}$$

Next, I determine the flow rate for the first 20 minutes.

Now I determine the flow rate to be used after the first 20 minutes.

$$X = 18 \text{ ml}$$

• After 20 minutes, reset the pump to deliver 18 ml/hour. That's 18 ml/60 minutes, or 0.3 ml/minute. Because there are 10 mU/ml, multiply 10 by 0.3 ml/minute to verify that this flow rate does provide 3 mU/minute.

Seizure? Stop it with magnesium sulfate.

Your patient is at risk for a seizure due to pregnancy-induced hypertension. The doctor orders *4 g (4,000 mg) magnesium sulfate in 250 ml D_5W to be infused at 2 g/hour.* What's the flow rate in milliliters per hour?
Here's one approach to solving this problem:
• Set up a proportion with the known concentration in one fraction and the flow rate in grams and the unknown flow rate in milliliters in the other fraction:

$$\frac{4 \text{ g}}{250 \text{ ml}} = \frac{2 \text{ g}}{X}$$

• Cross-multiply the fractions:

$$X \times 4 \text{ g} = 250 \text{ ml} \times 2 \text{ g}$$

• Solve for X by dividing each side of the equation by 4 g and canceling units that appear in both the numerator and denominator:

$$\frac{X \times 4\cancel{g}}{4\cancel{g}} = \frac{250 \text{ ml} \times 2 \cancel{g}}{4 \cancel{g}}$$

$$X = \frac{250 \text{ ml} \times 2}{4}$$

$$X = \frac{500 \text{ ml}}{4}$$

$$X = 125 \text{ ml}$$

The magnesium sulfate solution should be infused at 125 ml/hour.

Let's seize that problem again

Here's another approach to solving the same problem:
• First calculate the strength of the solution by setting up a proportion with the known strength in one fraction and the unknown strength in the other fraction:

$$\frac{4 \text{ g}}{250 \text{ ml}} = \frac{X}{1 \text{ ml}}$$

- Cross-multiply the fractions:

$$X \times 250 \text{ ml} = 4 \text{ g} \times 1 \text{ ml}$$

- Solve for X by dividing each side of the equation by 250 ml and canceling units that appear in both the numerator and denominator:

$$\frac{X \times 250 \text{ ml}}{250 \text{ ml}} = \frac{4 \text{ g} \times 1 \text{ ml}}{250 \text{ ml}}$$

$$X = \frac{4\text{g}}{250}$$

$$X = 0.016 \text{ g}$$

- The solution's strength is 0.016 g/ml. Next, calculate the flow rate by setting up another proportion with the solution concentration in one fraction and the unknown flow rate in the other fraction:

$$\frac{1 \text{ ml}}{0.016 \text{ g}} = \frac{X}{2 \text{ g}}$$

- Cross-multiply the fractions:

$$X \times 0.016 \text{ g} = 1 \text{ ml} \times 2 \text{ g}$$

- Solve for X by dividing each side of the equation by 0.016 g and canceling units that appear in both the numerator and denominator:

$$\frac{X \times 0.016 \text{ g}}{0.016 \text{ g}} = \frac{1 \text{ ml} \times 2 \text{ g}}{0.016 \text{ g}}$$

$$X = \frac{2 \text{ ml}}{0.016}$$

$$X = 125 \text{ ml}$$

The same flow rate of 125 ml per hour is obtained using this method.

Preterm labor? Try terbutaline.

Your patient is in preterm labor. The doctor prescribes *10 mg terbutaline sulfate in 250 ml of D₅W to infuse at 5 mcg/minute.* What's the flow rate for this solution?

Nothing feels better than getting the right answer twice!

- First, find the solution's strength. Set up a proportion with the known strength in one fraction and the unknown strength in the other fraction:

To begin, I calculate the solution's strength.

$$\frac{10 \text{ mg}}{250 \text{ ml}} = \frac{X \text{ mg}}{1 \text{ ml}}$$

- Cross-multiply the fractions:

$$X \text{ mg} \times 250 \text{ ml} = 10 \text{ mg} \times 1 \text{ ml}$$

- Solve for X by dividing each side of the equation by 250 ml and canceling units that appear in both the numerator and denominator:

$$\frac{X \times 250 \text{ ml}}{250 \text{ ml}} = \frac{10 \text{ mg} \times 1 \text{ ml}}{250 \text{ ml}}$$

$$X = \frac{10 \text{ mg}}{250}$$

$$X = .04 \text{ mg}$$

- The strength of the solution is 0.4 mg/ml. Next, convert to micrograms (mcg) by multiplying by 1,000 (.04 mg × 1,000 = 40 mcg/ml). Then calculate the flow rate needed to deliver the pre-scribed dose of 5 mcg/minute. To do this, set up a proportion with the known solution strength in one fraction and the unknown flow rate in the other:

$$\frac{1 \text{ ml}}{40 \text{ mcg}} = \frac{X}{5 \text{ mcg}}$$

Then I calculate the flow rate per minute.

- Cross-multiply the fractions:

$$X \times 40 \text{ mcg} = 1 \text{ ml} \times 5 \text{ mcg}$$

- Solve for X by dividing each side of the equation by 40 mcg and canceling units that appear in both the numerator and denominator:

$$\frac{X \times 40 \text{ mcg}}{40 \text{ mcg}} = \frac{1 \text{ ml} \times 5 \text{ mcg}}{40 \text{ mcg}}$$

$$X = \frac{5 \text{ mcg}}{40}$$

$$X = .125 \text{ ml}$$

- The flow rate is 0.125 ml/minute. Because the infusion must be administered with a pump, compute the hourly flow rate by set-ting up a proportion with the flow rate per minute in one fraction and the unknown flow rate in the other fraction:

$$\frac{0.125 \text{ ml}}{1 \text{ minute}} = \frac{X}{60 \text{ minutes}}$$

- Cross-multiply the fractions:

$$X \times 1 \text{ minute} = 0.125 \text{ ml} \times 60 \text{ minutes}$$

- Solve for X by dividing each side of the equation by 1 minute and canceling units that appear in both the numerator and denominator:

$$\frac{X \times 1 \text{ minute}}{1 \text{ minute}} = \frac{0.125 \text{ ml} \times 60 \text{ minutes}}{1 \text{ minute}}$$

$$X = 7.5 \text{ ml}$$

Round off the answer of 7.5 ml to the nearest milliliter, and set the infusion pump to deliver 8 ml/hour.

Last but not least, I calculate the hourly flow rate.

Quick quiz

1. If the order reads *20 U oxytocin (Pitocin) in 1,000 ml of lactated Ringer's solution*, the solution's concentration is:
    A.   20 U/ml.
    B.   2 U/ml.
    C.   0.02 U/ml.

Answer: A. To solve this problem, set up a proportion with the known concentration in one fraction and the unknown concentration in the other fraction. Then solve for X.

2. A sudden increase or decrease in the fetal heart rate after drug treatment is a :
    A.   sign that the infant is about to be delivered.
    B.   sign of an adverse reaction to the drug.
    C.   temporary reaction to many obstetric drugs.

Answer: B. If changes in the fetal heart rate occur, discontinue the drug immediately.

3. Which drug should be kept readily available to reverse magnesium sulfate intoxication?
    A.   potassium chloride
    B.   calcium gluconate
    C.   atropine

Answer: B. During magnesium sulfate infusion, calcium gluconate should be readily available to reverse magnesium intoxication should it occur.

4. If an order says *infuse 20 mg terbutaline sulfate in 1,000 ml of D_5W at 0.01 mg/minute for 20 minutes*, the flow rate should be:

    A.   1 ml.
    B.   10 ml.
    C.   100 ml.

Answer: B. First, calculate the concentration, which is 0.02 mg/ml. Then determine the amount of drug provided in 20 minutes by multiplying 0.01 by 20 minutes to get 0.2 mg. Finally, set up a proportion with the concentration in one fraction and the total amount of medication and the unknown flow rate in the other fraction. Solve for X to get 10 ml.

5. If 5 g of magnesium sulfate are added to 1 L of normal saline solution, the concentration of magnesium sulfate is:

    A.   5 mg/ml.
    B.   50 mg/ml.
    C.   0.05 mg/ml.

Answer: A. First, convert 5 g to 5,000 mg and 1 L to 1,000 ml. Then divide the 1,000 into 5,000 to obtain the concentration of the solution: 5 mg/ml.

6. If the doctor orders *20 g magnesium sulfate in 1,000 ml of D_5W to be infused at 5 g/hour*, the flow rate in milliliters per hour is:

    A.   2 ml/hour.
    B.   25 ml/hour.
    C.   250 ml/hour.

Answer: C. To solve this problem, set up a proportion with the ordered concentration in one fraction and the flow rate in grams and the unknown flow rate in milliliters in the other fraction. Solve for X.

7. The best way to administer oxytocin is:
A.   I.V. bolus injection.
B.   I.V. piggyback infusion.
C.   direct I.V. infusion.

Answer: B. Administer oxytocin by I.V. piggyback infusion using an infusion pump so that the drug can be discontinued without interrupting the I.V. line.

Scoring

☆☆☆ If you answered all seven items correctly, fantastic! Your labors have helped you become a confident calculator!

☆☆ If you answered five or six correctly, keep at it! You'll soon be able to deftly deliver drugs in any delivery unit!

☆ If you answered fewer than five correctly, you still have one chapter left to conquer the Quick Quiz!

15

Calculating critical care dosages

Just the facts

In this chapter, you'll learn:

♦ special points to consider when giving critical care drugs

♦ how to calculate dosages for I.V. push drugs

♦ how to calculate I.V. flow rates for critical care drugs

♦ how to calculate drugs not ordered at a specific flow rate or dosage.

In the critical care unit, dosage calculations need to be quick and accurate.

A look at critical care dosages

If you work on a critical care unit, you not only need to perform dosage calculations accurately, you also need to perform them quickly because of the patient's life-threatening condition. (See *Quick list of critical care meds and measurements*, page 270.)

Many I.V. drugs — such as the antiarrhythmics lidocaine and procainamide, the vasodilators sodium nitroprusside and nitroglycerin, and the adrenergics norepinephrine and dopamine — are administered in life-threatening situations. The nurse's job is to prepare the drug for infusion, give it to the patient, and then observe him to evaluate the drug's effectiveness.

Administering I.V. injections

Many drugs administered on critical care units are given by direct injection, also called I.V. push. These potent, fast-acting drugs rapidly control heart rate, respirations, blood pressure, cardiac output, or kidney function. They usually have a short duration of action, so you can evaluate their effectiveness immediately and begin other treatment promptly if they aren't working.

One critical difference

Generally, the doctor orders I.V. push drugs by dosage, which can sometimes include mg/minute. Calculate dosages on the critical care unit the same as you would on other units. However, take extra care because drugs used on critical care units are extremely potent and have serious adverse effects, which can include death.

Be prepared to be under stress

You're responsible for calculating and administering the dose accurately, following any special instructions. Many drugs used on critical care units come in small vials, so double-check the label to make sure you're giving the right dose or concentration. For example, epinephrine comes in two concentrations (1:1,000 and 1:10,000). Giving the wrong concentration could be fatal.

Because calculating dosages during an emergency is stressful, and stress makes you more error-prone, do everything you can to be prepared. (See *Stress busters.*)

Calculating dosages

The following examples demonstrate how to use proportions to calculate I.V. push drugs. Note that the calculations are very similar to those for intramuscular (I.M.) drugs.

Also note how the administration times vary. If you aren't sure how slowly or quickly to push a drug, look it up or call the pharmacist. It's better to be safe than sorry with rapid-acting drugs.

Are you label able?

Your patient is admitted with frequent ventricular arrhythmias. The doctor orders *procainamide 200 mg q 5 min by slow I.V. push (no faster than 25 to 50 mg/minute) until arrhythmias disappear.* If the drug label says to administer 100 mg/ml, how many milliliters of procainamide should you give to the patient every five minutes? (See *Procainamide label.*)

• Set up a proportion with the ordered dose and the unknown dose in one fraction and the dose in milligrams per milliliter in the other fraction:

$$\frac{200 \text{ mg}}{X} = \frac{100 \text{ mg}}{1 \text{ ml}}$$

• Cross-multiply the fractions:

$$X \times 100 \text{ mg} = 1 \text{ ml} \times 200 \text{ mg}$$

I can't waste time

Quick list of critical care meds and measurements

The list below shows some of the common critical care drugs and associated units of measure. Memorizing these units of measure will help speed your calculations:

• epinephrine: mcg/minute
• nitroglycerin: mg/minute
• norepinephrine: mcg/minute
• phenylephrine: mcg/minute
• nitroprusside: mcg/kg/minute
• dopamine: mcg/kg/minute
• dobutamine: mcg/kg/minute
• procainamide: mg/minute
• lidocaine: mg/minute.

- Solve for X by dividing each side of the equation by 100 mg and canceling the units that appear in both the numerator and denominator:

$$\frac{X \times \cancel{100 \text{ mg}}}{\cancel{100 \text{ mg}}} = \frac{1 \text{ ml} \times 200 \cancel{\text{ mg}}}{100 \cancel{\text{ mg}}}$$

$$X = \frac{200 \text{ ml}}{100}$$

$$X = 2 \text{ ml}$$

You should administer 2 ml, or one-fifth of the contents of the procainamide vial. According to the package insert, you should administer the drug only I.M. or I.V. Also note that when giving procainamide I.V., the drug must be diluted.

Rapid heartbeat riddle

Your patient suddenly develops supraventricular tachycardia. The doctor orders *6 mg adenosine rapid I.V. push.* If the only vial available contains 3 mg/ml, how many milliliters should you give?
- Set up a proportion with the available solution in one ratio and the ordered dose and the unknown dose in the other ratio:

$$3 \text{ mg} : 1 \text{ ml} :: 6 \text{ mg} : X$$

- Multiply the means and the extremes:

$$X \times 3 \text{ mg} = 1 \text{ ml} \times 6 \text{ mg}$$

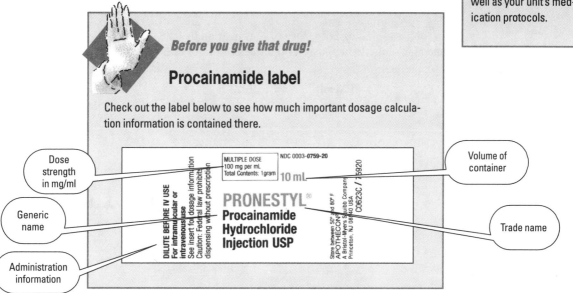

Before you give that drug!

Procainamide label

Check out the label below to see how much important dosage calculation information is contained there.

Dose strength in mg/ml

Generic name

Administration information

Volume of container

Trade name

MULTIPLE DOSE
100 mg per mL
Total Contents: 1gram

NDC 0003-**0759-20**

10 mL

DILUTE BEFORE IV USE
For intramuscular or intravenous use
See insert for dosage information
Caution: Federal law prohibits dispensing without prescription

PRONESTYL®
Procainamide Hydrochloride Injection USP

Store between 59° and 80° F
APOTHECON®
A Bristol-Myers Squibb Company
Princeton, NJ 08540 USA

C0623C / 75920

• Solve for X by dividing both sides of the equation by 3 mg and canceling units that appear in both the numerator and denominator:

$$\frac{X \times 3\ \cancel{mg}}{3\ \cancel{mg}} = \frac{1\ ml \times 6\ \cancel{mg}}{3\ \cancel{mg}}$$

$$X = \frac{6\ ml}{3}$$

$$X = 2\ ml$$

You should administer 2 ml of the solution. According to the package insert, this drug should be administered by rapid I.V. push because of its very short half-life. It also should be administered directly into the vein or in the most proximal port, followed by a rapid saline flush.

Digoxin difficulty

Your patient has a history of rapid atrial fibrillation and takes digoxin at home. When his digoxin level is found to be subtherapeutic, the doctor orders *0.125 mg I.V digoxin as a single dose* to control his heart rate. The only available digoxin vial contains 0.25 mg/ml. How many milliliters should you give?

• Set up a proportion with the available solution in one ratio and the ordered dose and the unknown dose in the other ratio:

$$0.25\ mg : 1\ ml :: 0.125\ mg : X$$

• Multiply the means and the extremes:

$$X \times 0.25\ mg = 1\ ml \times 0.125\ mg$$

• Solve for X by dividing both sides of the equation by 0.25 mg and canceling units that appear in both the numerator and denominator:

$$\frac{X \times 0.25\ \cancel{mg}}{0.25\ \cancel{mg}} = \frac{1\ ml \times 0.125\ \cancel{mg}}{0.25\ \cancel{mg}}$$

$$X = \frac{0.125\ ml}{0.25}$$

$$X = 0.5\ ml$$

You should administer 0.5 ml of digoxin. According to the package insert, give it by I.V. push over 5 minutes.

Calculating I.V. flow rates

Because many drugs given on the critical care unit are used to treat life-threatening problems, you can't waste time calculating I.V. flow rates. You must swiftly do the calculations, prepare the drug for infusion, administer it, and then observe the patient closely to evaluate the drug's effectiveness.

Cheat sheet

Concentration formula

- *Concentration in mg/ml:* mg of drug ÷ ml of fluid

Three critical calculations

You may need to perform three calculations before administering critical care drugs:

 concentration of the drug in the I.V. solution

flow rate required to deliver the desired dose

 number of micrograms needed, based on the patient's weight in kilograms. You may need to perform this calculation if the drug is ordered in micrograms per kilogram of body weight per minute. *Remember:* If you need to convert milligrams to micrograms, multiply by 1,000.

Concentrate on this formula

To calculate the drug's concentration, use the following formula:

$$\text{concentration in mg/ml} = \frac{\text{mg of drug}}{\text{ml of fluid}}$$

- If you need to express the concentration in mcg/ml, multiply the answer by 1,000.

Figuring flow rate

You can determine the I.V. flow rate per minute, using the following formula:

$$\frac{\text{dose/minute}}{X} = \frac{\text{concentration of solution}}{1 \text{ ml of fluid}}$$

- To calculate the hourly flow rate, first multiply the ordered dose, given in milligrams or micrograms per minute, by 60 minutes to determine the hourly dose. Then use the following proportion to compute the hourly flow rate:

$$\frac{\text{hourly dose}}{X} = \frac{\text{concentration of solution}}{1 \text{ ml of fluid}}$$

Determining the dosage

To determine the dosage in milligrams per kilogram of body weight per minute, perform the following steps:
• First, determine the concentration of the solution in milligrams per milliliter. To determine the dose in milligrams per hour, multiply the hourly flow rate by the concentration using the formula:

$$\text{dose in mg/hour} = \text{hourly flow rate} \times \text{concentration}$$

• To calculate the dose in milligrams per minute, first divide the hourly dose by 60 minutes. Here's the formula:

$$\text{dose in mg/minute} = \frac{\text{dose in mg/hour}}{60 \text{ minutes}}$$

• Then divide the dose per minute by the patient's weight, using this formula:

$$\text{mg/kg/minute} = \frac{\text{mg/minute}}{\text{patient's weight in kg}}$$

• Once you've performed these calculations, make sure that the drug is being given within a safe and therapeutic range. Compare the amount in milligrams per kilogram per minute to the safe range shown in a drug reference book. (See *No time for books?*)

Real world problems

The following examples show how to calculate an I.V. flow rate using the different formulas.

Don't miss a beat

Your patient is having frequent runs of ventricular tachycardia that subside after 10 to 12 beats. The doctor orders *2 g (2,000 mg) lidocaine in 500 ml of D₅W to infuse at 2 mg/minute.* What's the flow rate in milliliters per minute? In milliliters per hour?
• First, find the solution's concentration by setting up a proportion with the unknown concentration in one fraction and the ordered dose in the other fraction:

$$\frac{X}{1 \text{ ml}} = \frac{2,000 \text{ mg}}{500 \text{ ml}}$$

• Cross-multiply the fractions:

$$X \times 500 \text{ ml} = 2,000 \text{ mg} \times 1 \text{ ml}$$

First, I determine the solution's concentration.

I can't waste time

No time for books?

Suppose you don't have time to refer to your dosage calculation book in a critical situation. Keep these formulas on a card with your calculator for quick reference. They're foolproof!

• To find out how many micrograms per kilogram per minute your patient is receiving, use this formula:

$$\frac{mg}{\text{volume of bag}} \times 1000 \div 60 \div kg \times \text{infusion rate} = \text{mcg/kg/min}$$

• To find out how many milliliters per hour you should give, use this formula:

$$\frac{\text{weight in kg} \times \text{dose in mcg/kg/min} \times 60}{\text{concentration in 1L}} = \text{ml/hr}$$

• Solve for X by dividing each side of the equation by 500 ml and canceling units that appear in both the numerator and denominator:

$$\frac{X \times 500\ \cancel{ml}}{500\ \cancel{ml}} = \frac{2,000\ mg \times 1\ \cancel{ml}}{500\ \cancel{ml}}$$

$$X = \frac{2,000\ mg}{500}$$

$$X = 4\ mg$$

• The solution's concentration is 4 mg/ml. Next, calculate the flow rate per minute needed to deliver the ordered dose of 2 mg/minute. To do this, set up a proportion with the unknown flow rate per minute in one fraction and the solution's concentration in the other fraction:

$$\frac{2\ mg}{X} = \frac{4\ mg}{1\ ml}$$

• Cross-multiply the fractions:

$$X \times 4\ mg = 1\ ml \times 2\ mg$$

Next, I calculate the flow rate per minute.

- Solve for X by dividing each side of the equation by 4 mg and canceling units that appear in both the numerator and denominator:

$$\frac{X \times 4\,\cancel{mg}}{4\,\cancel{mg}} = \frac{1 \text{ ml} \times 2\,\cancel{mg}}{4\,\cancel{mg}}$$

$$X = \frac{2 \text{ ml}}{4}$$

$$X = 0.5 \text{ ml}$$

- The patient should receive 0.5 ml/minute of lidocaine. Because lidocaine must be infused through an infusion pump, compute the hourly flow rate. Do this by setting up a proportion with the unknown flow rate per hour in one fraction and the flow rate per minute in the other fraction:

$$\frac{X}{60 \text{ minutes}} = \frac{0.5 \text{ ml}}{1 \text{ minute}}$$

- Cross-multiply the fractions:

$$X \times 1 \text{ minute} = 0.5 \text{ ml} \times 60 \text{ minutes}$$

- Solve for X by dividing each side of the equation by 1 minute and canceling units that appear in both the numerator and denominator:

$$\frac{X \times 1\,\cancel{\text{minute}}}{1\,\cancel{\text{minute}}} = \frac{0.5 \text{ ml} \times 60\,\cancel{\text{minutes}}}{1\,\cancel{\text{minute}}}$$

$$X = 30 \text{ ml}$$

Set the infusion pump to deliver 30 ml/hour.

Computing after diluting

A 200-lb patient is to receive an I.V. infusion of dobutamine at 10 mcg/kg/minute. The label says to check the package insert. There it says to dilute 250 mg of the drug in 50 ml of D_5W. (See *Dobutamine label.*)

Because the drug vial contains 20 ml of solution, the total to be infused is 70 ml (50 ml of D_5W + 20 ml of solution). How many milliliters of the drug should the patient receive each minute? Each hour?

- First, compute the patient's weight in kilograms. To do this, set up a proportion with the weight in pounds and the unknown

First, compute the patient's weight in kilograms.

weight in kilograms in one fraction and the number of pounds per kilogram in the other fraction:

$$\frac{200 \text{ lb}}{X} = \frac{2.2 \text{ lb}}{1 \text{ kg}}$$

• Cross-multiply the fractions:

$$X \times 2.2 \text{ lb} = 1 \text{ kg} \times 200 \text{ lb}$$

• Solve for X by dividing each side of the equation by 2.2 lb and canceling units that appear in both the numerator and denominator:

$$\frac{X \times 2.2 \cancel{\text{ lb}}}{2.2 \cancel{\text{ lb}}} = \frac{1 \text{ kg} \times 200 \cancel{\text{ lb}}}{2.2 \cancel{\text{ lb}}}$$

$$X = \frac{200 \text{ kg}}{2.2}$$

$$X = 90.9 \text{ kg}$$

• The patient weighs 90.9 kg. Next, determine the dose in milliliters per minute by setting up a proportion with the patient's weight in kilograms and the unknown dose in micrograms per

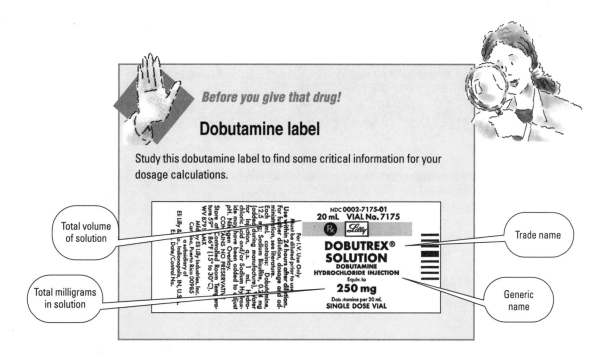

Before you give that drug!

Dobutamine label

Study this dobutamine label to find some critical information for your dosage calculations.

Total volume of solution

Total milligrams in solution

Trade name

Generic name

minute in one fraction and the known dose in micrograms per kilogram per minute in the other fraction:

$$\frac{90.9 \text{ kg}}{X} = \frac{1 \text{ kg}}{10 \text{ mcg/minute}}$$

Next, I determine the dose in mcg/minute.

- Cross-multiply the fractions:

$$X \times 1 \text{ kg} = 10 \text{ mcg/minute} \times 90.9 \text{ kg}$$

- Solve for X by dividing each side of the equation by 1 kg and canceling units that appear in both the numerator and denominator:

$$\frac{X \times \cancel{1 \text{ kg}}}{\cancel{1 \text{ kg}}} = \frac{10 \text{ mcg/minute} \times 90.9 \cancel{\text{ kg}}}{1 \cancel{\text{ kg}}}$$

$$X = 909 \text{ mcg/minute}$$

- The patient should receive 909 mcg of dobutamine every minute. To determine the flow rate in milliliters per minute, set up a proportion using the solution's concentration and solve for X:

$$\frac{0.909 \text{ mg}}{X} = \frac{3.6 \text{ mg}}{1 \text{ ml}}$$

$$X = \frac{0.909}{3.6}$$

$$X = 0.2525 \text{ ml/minute}$$

Finally, I calculate the dose in ml/hour.

- To find the flow rate in milliliters per hour, multiply by 60.

$$0.2525 \text{ ml/minute} \times 60 \text{ minutes/hour} = 15.15 \text{ ml/hour}$$

The patient should receive dobutamine at a rate of 15 ml/hr.

Special cases

Critical care drugs aren't always ordered at a specific flow rate or dosage. Sometimes, they're prescribed according to the patient's heart rate, blood pressure, or other parameters.

In some cases, the doctor may order a starting dose and a maximum dose to which the drug can be titrated. To deliver the correct amount of drug, you must calculate the starting dose and the maximum dose.

Here are some examples of drug calculations that you may use in special cases.

Nitroprusside number cruncher

A patient with severe hypertension weighs 85 kg. The doctor's order reads *nitroprusside 50 mg in 250 ml of D₅W. Start at 0.5 mcg/kg/minute. Titrate to keep systolic BP < 170 mm Hg. Maximum dose is 5 mcg/kg/minute*. At what rate should you start the infusion?

- First find the concentration of the infusion. Start by converting 50 mg to 50,000 mcg.

$$\frac{50,000 \text{ mcg}}{250 \text{ ml}} = 200 \text{ mcg/ml}$$

- Then set up the following equation:

$$X = \frac{85 \text{ kg} \times 0.5 \text{ mcg/kg/min} \times 60}{200 \text{ mcg/ml}}$$

$$X = 12.75 \text{ ml/hr}$$

The starting dose is 13 ml/hour.

In this case, I need to make sure the maximum dose for this patient isn't exceeded!

Determine this saline solution

A patient with terminal Hodgkin's disease who weighs 90 lb (41 kg) has been hypotensive for several hours despite receiving I.V. fluid boluses. The doctor orders *100 mg phenylephrine in 250 ml of normal saline solution*. The drug is to start at 30 mcg/minute and then be titrated to keep the systolic blood pressure at 90 mm Hg. What's the flow rate in milliliters per minute?

- First, determine the solution's concentration by dividing the ordered dose of phenylephrine by the amount of normal saline solution:

$$X = \frac{100 \text{ mg}}{250 \text{ ml}}$$

$$X = 0.4 \text{ mg/ml}$$

- The concentration is 0.4 mg/ml. Next, convert milligrams to micrograms by multiplying by 1,000:

$$0.4 \text{ mg/ml} \times 1,000 = 400 \text{ mcg/ml}$$

- The concentration is 400 mcg/ml. Now, calculate the flow rate by setting up a proportion with the starting flow rate and the unknown flow rate in one fraction and the concentration in the other fraction:

First, determine the concentration.

$$\frac{30 \text{ mcg/minute}}{X \text{ ml/minute}} = \frac{400 \text{ mcg}}{1 \text{ ml}}$$

- Cross-multiply the fractions:

$$X \text{ ml/minute} \times 400 \text{ mcg} = 30 \text{ mcg/minute} \times 1 \text{ ml}$$

- Solve for X by dividing each side of the equation by 400 mcg and canceling units that appear in both the numerator and denominator:

$$\frac{X \text{ ml/minute} \times \cancel{400 \text{ mcg}}}{\cancel{400 \text{ mcg}}} = \frac{30 \cancel{\text{ mcg}}\text{/minute} \times 1 \text{ ml}}{400 \cancel{\text{ mcg}}}$$

$$X = \frac{30 \text{ ml/minute}}{400}$$

$$X = 0.075 \text{ ml/minute}$$

- The flow rate is 0.075 ml/minute. To calculate the hourly flow rate, multiply 0.075 ml by 60:

$$0.075 \text{ ml} \times 60 = 4.5 \text{ ml}$$

The hourly flow rate is 4.5 ml, which can be rounded off to 5 ml/hour.

Finally, I find the hourly flow rate!

Quick quiz

1. If a patient has a dopamine drip of 800 mg in 500 ml of D_5W, the concentration is:

    A.   0.16 mg/ml.
    B.   1.6 mg/ml.
    C.   160 mg/ml.

Answer: B. Concentration is determined by dividing the total in milligrams (800 mg) by the volume (500 ml).

2. Procainamide is measured in:

    A.   mcg/kg/minute.
    B.   mg/minute.
    C.   mg/hour.

Answer: B. This information is necessary before you can calculate dosages of procainamide.

3. To convert milligrams to micrograms, multiply by:

    A.   60.

B.   10.
C.   1,000.

Answer: C. When converting a number from milligrams to micrograms, move the decimal three spaces to the right.

4.   How many kilograms does a 250-lb man weigh?
   A.   114 kg
   B.   11.4 kg
   C.   550 kg

Answer: A. To convert pounds to kilograms, divide by 2.2 and
round off the number.

5.   The doctor's order reads *Lasix 80 mg I.V. as a single dose.*
The available vial contains 100 mg in 10 ml of normal saline solu-
tion. What volume should you give to accomplish this dose?
   A.   0.8 ml
   B.   8 ml
   C.   0.08 ml

Answer: B. Set up a proportion with the available solution in one
ratio and the ordered dose and the unknown volume in the other
ratio. Solve for *X*.

Five down,
two to go!

6. If a patient weighs 50 kg, his weight in pounds is:
   A.   110 lb.
   B.   200 lb.
   C.   28 lb.

Answer: A. To convert kilograms to pounds, multiply by 2.2.

7. A patient requires nitroprusside to lower his blood pressure. This dose should be ordered in:
   A.   mcg/kg/minute
   B.   mcg/minute
   C.   mg/minute

Answer: A. Nitroprusside should be ordered in doses of mcg/kg/minute.

Scoring

☆☆☆ If you answered all seven items correctly, fantastic! You can calculate confidently in critical cases!

☆☆ If you answered five or six correctly, that isn't bad! You're a cool, calm, and collected calculator!

☆ If you answered fewer than five correctly, keep at it! You have the best dosage calc book ever! Keep it with you always and refer to it frequently.

Appendices and index

Practice makes perfect   284

Glossary   302

Index   305

Practice makes perfect

1. The improper fraction $^{11}\!/_2$ converted into a mixed number is:
    A. $^2\!/_{11}$.
    B. $5^1\!/_{11}$.
    Ⓒ $5^1\!/_2$.

2. The sum of $^1\!/_2 + {}^3\!/_4 + {}^6\!/_{10}$ equals:
    A. $1^8\!/_{10}$.
    B. $1^{17}\!/_{20}$.
    C. $2^1\!/_4$.

3. The complex fraction $^1\!/_{75}$ divided by the complex fraction $^1\!/_{25}$ equals:
    A. $^1\!/_3$.
    B.   3.
    C. $^1\!/_{100}$.

4. The decimal fraction 4.3 divided by 8.6 yields:
    A.   0.5.
    B.   2.
    C.   20.

5. When 21.3478 is rounded off to the nearest hundredth, it becomes:
    A.   21.34.
    B.   21.35.
    C.   21.348.

6. 31% of 105 is:
    A.   3.15.
    B.   31.5.
    C.   32.55.

7. When 20% is converted to a decimal fraction, it becomes:
    A.   0.02.
    B.   2.0.
    C.   0.2.

8. In fraction form, the proportion 1 : 4 :: 4 : 16 is:
    A. $4/1 = 4/16$.
    B. $1/4 = 4/16$.
    C. $4/4 = 1/16$.

9. If a vial has 20 mg of drug in 50 ml of solution, the amount of drug in 10 ml of solution is:
    A.   4 mg
    B.   10 mg
    C.   5 mg

10. In the proportion $3 : 9 :: 9 : X. X$ equals:
    A.   81.
    B.   3.
    C.   27.

11. How much chlorine bleach should you add to 500 ml of water to make a solution that contains 10 ml of chlorine bleach for every 100 ml of water?
    A.   5 ml
    B.   50 ml
    C.   10 ml

12. A patient weighs 70 kg. How many pounds is this?
- A. 140 lb
- B. 154 lb
- C. 70 lb

13. A patient has been ordered *ampicillin 250 mg*. The medication is supplied as an oral suspension, 125 mg per 5 ml. How many milliliters should the patient receive?
- A. 10 ml
- B. 5 ml
- C. 1 ml

14. The doctor prescribes meperidine 75 mg. The pharmacy stocks a multidose vial containing 100 mg/ml. How many milliliters should you administer?
- A. 7.5 ml
- B. 0.75 ml
- C. 0.25 ml

15. Convert 0.025 kl to L.
- A. 250 L
- B. 2.5 L
- C. 25 L

16. During a 24-hour period, a patient received 600 ml, 1.25 L, and 2.5 L of I.V. fluid. How many milliliters did he receive all together?
- A. 43,500 ml
- B. 43.5 ml
- C. 4350 ml

17. The weight in kilograms of a baby that weighs 8,300 g is:
- A. 8,300 kg
- B. 8.3 kg
- C. 83.0 kg

18. A patient receives 0.25 mg of digoxin (Lanoxin). How many grams did he receive?

    A.   25 g

    B.   00025 g

    C.   0.25 g

19. According to the medication order, a patient is to receive 2 gr of a drug. The bottle is labeled 120 mg/ml. How many milliliters will you give?

    A.   1 ml

    B.   2 ml

    C.   30 ml

20. A patient's fingerstick glucose level was 365 mg/dl. The doctor has ordered 10 U of regular insulin for the patient. The bottle is labeled 100 U/ml. The volume of insulin you'll administer is:

    A.   0.01 ml.

    B.   0.1 ml.

    C.   1.0 ml.

21. A patient needs 20 mEq of potassium chloride oral solution. The solution contains 60 mEq in every 15 ml. How many milliliters of solution should you give the patient?

    A.   5 ml

    B.   2.5 ml

    C.   7.5 ml

22. The Arabic numeral 148 in Roman numerals is:

    A.   CLXVIII.

    B.   CXXXIIIIIIII.

    C.   DLXVIII.

23. A doctor prescribes *digoxin 0.125 mg P.O. 0900 qd* for a patient with heart failure. How should you interpret this order?
    A.   Give 125 grams of digoxin orally at 9 a.m. every other day.
    B.   Give 0.125 milligrams of digoxin orally every day at 9 p.m.
    C.   Give 0.125 milligrams of digoxin orally every day at 9 a.m.

24. Which of the following doctor's orders is incomplete?
    A.   *Tylenol elixir 1 tsp P.O. STAT*
    B.   *Aspirin 325 P.O. q a.m.*
    C.   *Seconal 100 mg P.O. h.s. p.r.n.*

25. The doctor prescribes *nifedipine 300 mg SL q4h* for a patient with hypertension. You should understand that this drug is to be given:
    A.   four times per day.
    B.   in a suspension.
    C.   under the tongue.

26. You're administering medication to a 58-year-old patient who was admitted with heart failure. In giving a regularly scheduled drug, you must:
    A.   give the drug one-half hour before or after the ordered time.
    B.   give the drug 1 hour before or after the ordered time.
    C.   give the drug 15 minutes before or after the ordered time.

27. You need to administer morphine to a patient who just returned from the postanesthesia care unit after undergoing a laminectomy. The information recorded on the perpetual inventory record when you remove a controlled substance from a locked storage site should include:
    A.   date and time of removal, patient's name, drug dose, and your initials.
    B.   date and time of removal, patient's name, drug dose, and your signature.
    C.   date and time of removal, patient's name, doctor's name, drug dose, and your signature.

28. You're caring for a 49-year-old patient with metastatic breast cancer. You need to administer her 9 a.m. medications. When administering regularly scheduled drugs, you should:

    A.   document the time of administration prior to giving the drug to the patient.

    B.   document the time of administration after giving the drug to the patient.

    C.   document the time of administration for all regularly scheduled drugs on your shift at the beginning of the shift.

29. A patient tells you that she typically takes two ibuprofen tablets for menstrual cramps. If one tablet of ibuprofen contains 200 mg, how many milligrams does she usually take?

    A.   500 mg

    B.   600 mg

    C.   400 mg

30. Before administering a patient's medication, you should compare the drug ordered with the drug's label. The nonproprietary name on a drug label is:

    A.   trade name.

    B.   generic name.

    C.   manufacturer name.

31. The doctor orders *minoxidil 5 mg P.O. daily* for treatment of hypertension in a 52-year-old patient. The medication is supplied as 2.5 mg per tablet. How many tablets should be administered?

    A.   2 tablets

    B.   ½ tablet

    C.   2½ tablets

32. An 83-year-old patient complains that she hasn't had a bowel movement for 4 days and she's very uncomfortable. The doctor orders *Milk of Magnesia 1½ tsp P.O. h.s.* How many milliliters is this?

    A.   17.5 ml

    B.   15.5 ml

    C.   22.5 ml

33. A patient is ordered *Tylenol 240 mg supp per rectum* to treat a fever. You have Tylenol 120 mg supp available. What should be prepared?

    A.   1½ supp
    B.   1 supp
    C.   2 supp

34. A pediatric patient is ordered *Compazine 2.5 mg supp per rectum STAT* for treatment of postoperative nausea. Compazine 5 mg per supp is available. How much should be given?

    A.   ½ supp
    B.   1 supp
    C.   2 supp

35. A patient is ordered bacitracin for treatment of a wound he received in a motor vehicle crash. Before giving the patient a topical preparation, it's important to read the label first because:

    A.   you want to know the manufacturer's name.
    B.   the patient may be allergic to the ingredients.
    C.   you like to read small print.

36. A 52-year-old patient requires transdermal nitroglycerin to control his angina. You know that transdermal nitroglycerin should be removed 12 to 14 hours after application to:

    A.   prevent it falling off while the patient sleeps.
    B.   prevent it from irritating the patient's skin.
    C.   prevent the patient from developing a tolerance to the drug.

37. A patient returns from the postanesthesia care unit after undergoing an exploratory laparotomy and a lysis of adhesions. The doctor orders *Demerol 75 mg I.M. q4h p.r.n.* for pain. The medication is available in a prefilled syringe containing 100 mg of Demerol per 1 ml. How many milliliters of Demerol should you administer?

    A.   1 ml
    B.   0.75 ml
    C.   0.25 ml

38. The doctor orders *Dilaudid 3 mg I.M. q6h p.r.n.* for pain for a patient with postoperative pain. The medication is available in a pre-filled syringe containing 4 mg per ml. How many milliliters of Dilaudid should you waste?

    A.   0.25 ml

    B.   0.75 ml

    C.   0.5 ml

39. The doctor orders *heparin 8,000 U S.C. q8h* for a patient with deep vein thrombosis. The heparin available is 20,000 units per 1 ml. How many milliliters of heparin should you give?

    A.   0.2 ml

    B.   0.3 ml

    C.   0.4 ml

40. A patient with type 1 diabetes mellitus is ordered 45 U of NPH insulin subcutaneously in the morning daily. You have NPH insulin 100 U per ml available. Using a U-100 syringe, how many milliliters will be in the syringe?

    A.   0.045 ml

    B.   0.45 ml

    C.   4.5 ml

41. A patient needs an infusion of D_5W at 100 ml/hour. If the tubing set is calibrated at 15 gtt/ml, what's the drip rate?

    A.   31 gtt/minute

    B.   33 gtt/minute

    C.   25 gtt/minute

42. A patient diagnosed with pneumonia needs 2,000 ml of fluid over 24 hours. What's the flow rate?

    A.   83 ml/hour

    B.   100 ml/hour

    C.   125 ml/hour

43. You're about to administer a continuous infusion of 25,000 U of heparin in 500 ml of half-normal saline solution. If the patient is to receive 750 U/hour, what's the flow rate?
    A.   25 ml/hour
    B.   15 ml/hour
    C.   10 ml/hour

44. A 4-year-old patient weighs 46 lb. How many kilograms is this?
    A.   21 kg
    B.   20 kg
    C.   23 kg

45. The doctor orders a single dose of acetaminophen 10 mg/kg/dose oral suspension for a child with a fever who weighs 6 kg. What's the dose in milligrams?
    A.   1.6 mg
    B.   16 mg
    C.   60 mg

46. A child weighing 66 lb is admitted with appendicitis. How much maintenance I.V. fluid should the child receive in 24 hours.
    A.   1,500 ml/day
    B.   1,700 ml/day
    C.   1,800 ml/day

47. A 25-year-old primagravida has been in labor for 20 hours with little progress. The doctor prescribes oxytocin for her. The order reads *10 U oxytocin in 1,000 ml NSS to infuse via pump at 1 mU/minute for 15 minutes; then increase flow rate to 2 mU/ minute.* What's the flow rate needed to deliver 1 mU/minute for 15 minutes.
    A.   4 ml/hour
    B.   8 ml/hour
    C.   12 ml/hour

48. Use the calculations in the previous problem. After 15 minutes, the pump needs to be reset to deliver 2 mU/minute. What's the flow rate?

    A.   10 ml/hour

    B.   20 ml/hour

    C.   12 ml/hour

49. The doctor orders *4 g magnesium sulfate in 250 ml D$_5$W infused at 1 g/hour* for a patient with preeclampsia. What's the flow rate?

    A.   125 ml/hour

    B.   250 ml/hour

    C.   63 ml/hour

50. The doctor orders *150 mg of ritodrine hydrochloride in 500 ml D$_5$W to infuse at 0.15 mg/minute* for a patient admitted in preterm labor. What's the flow rate?

    A.   30 ml/hour

    B.   15 ml/hour

    C.   10 ml/hour

51. A 170-lb patient with minimal urine output has an order to receive dopamine at 5 mcg/kg/minute. The premixed bag of dopamine contains 800 mg in 500 ml D$_5$W. How many milliliters of solution containing dopamine will the patient receive each hour?

    A.   14 ml

    B.   15 ml

    C.   16 ml

52. A patient experiencing an acute myocardial infarction is to receive nitroglycerin 10 mcg/minute I.V. The I.V. solution contains 250 ml D$_5$W with 25 mg nitroglycerin. How many milliliters should the patient receive each hour?

    A.   16 ml

    B.   10 ml

    C.   6 ml

53. A patient experienced a sustained ventricular tachycardia that required cardioversion. The doctor orders *1 g lidocaine in 250 ml D_5W to infuse at 3 mg/minute.* to help maintain a normal sinus rhythm. What's the flow rate?

      A.   30 ml/hour
      B.   45 ml/hour
      C.   60 ml/hour

Answers

1.   C. Divide the numerator (11) by the denominator (2). The calculation looks like this:

$$\frac{11}{2} = 11 \div 2 = 5\tfrac{1}{2}$$

You get 5 with 1 left over. The 1 becomes the new numerator and the denominator stays the same.

2.   B. Determine the lowest common denominator (20). Then convert each to the lowest common denominator: $\frac{1}{2} = \frac{10}{20}$, $\frac{3}{4} = \frac{15}{20}$, $\frac{6}{10} = \frac{12}{20}$. Add all the numerators and place over the denominators: $\frac{10}{20} + \frac{15}{20} + \frac{12}{20} = \frac{37}{20}$. Reduce to lowest terms: $1\frac{17}{20}$.

3.   A. Divide the dividend $\frac{1}{75}$ by the divisor $\frac{1}{25}$. Invert the divisor ($\frac{1}{25}$) and multiply $\frac{1}{75} \times \frac{25}{1} = \frac{25}{75}$. Reduce to lowest terms: $\frac{1}{3}$.

4.   A. Move the decimal points of both the divisor and the dividend one place to the right before dividing. Place the quotient's decimal point over the new decimal point in the dividend.

5.   B. The number 4 is in the hundredth place. Look at the number to the right of it, which is 7. Seven is greater than 5 so add 1 to 4 to round off the number.

6.   C. To solve this, restate the question as a decimal fraction by removing the percent sign and moving the decimal point two places to the left. (The decimal fraction is 0.31.) Then multiply 0.31 by 105.

7.   C. Remove the percent sign and move the decimal point two places to the left.

8.   B. Make the ratio on both sides into fractions by substituting slashes for colons; replace the double colon in the center with an equal sign.

9. A. Substitute X for the amount of drug in 10 ml of solution; then set up a proportion with ratios or fractions:

$$X : 10 \text{ ml} = 20 \text{ mg} : 50 \text{ ml} \quad or \quad \frac{X}{10 \text{ ml}} = \frac{20 \text{ mg}}{50 \text{ ml}}$$

10. C. Multiply the means and the extremes. Put the products of the means and extremes into an equation. Solve for X by dividing both sides by 3. The calculation looks like this:

$$9 \times 9 = 3 \times X$$

$$81 = 3X$$

$$X = 27$$

11. B. Substitute X for the amount of chlorine bleach in 500 ml of water. Then set up a proportion with ratios or fractions. The set up looks like this:

X ml bleach/500 ml of water = 10 ml bleach/100 ml water

or

X ml bleach : 500 ml water :: 10 ml bleach : 100 ml water

12. B. Use the conversion factor 1 kg equals 2.2 lb to find that 70 kg equals 154 lb.

13. A. Use the conversion factor 125 mg equals 5 ml to find that the patient should receive 10 ml.

14. B. Set up the following equation and solve for X (X represents the milliliters needed to administer 75 mg.):

$$X = \frac{1 \text{ ml}}{100 \text{ mg}} \times \frac{75 \text{ mg}}{1}$$

15. C. Using the *Amazing metric decimal place finder*, page 82, count the number of places to the right or left of kiloliters to reach liters. In this case, it's three places to the right, so move the decimal three places to the right.

16. C. Knowing that there are 1,000 ml in 1 L, convert all the measurements to milliliters and add all the numbers together.

17. B. Knowing that 1 kg equals 1,000 g, set up an equation with X as the unknown quantity:

$$\frac{X}{0.25 \text{ mg}} = \frac{1 \text{ g}}{1000 \text{ mg}}$$

Cross-multiply and then divide both sides of the equation by 1,000 g to isolate X, canceling like units. Finish solving for X.

18. B. Using the *Insta-metric conversion table*, page 81, you'll see that 1 g is equal to 1,000 mg. Set up the equation with X as the unknown quantity:

$$\frac{X}{0.25\text{ mg}} = \frac{1\text{ g}}{1,000\text{ mg}}$$

Cross-multiply and then divide both sides of the equation by 1,000 mg to isolate X, canceling like units. Finish the math.

19. A. The known equivalent is 60 mg equals 1 gr. Set up an equation to determine how many milligrams there are in 2 grains by solving for X as the unknown quantity:

$$\frac{X}{2\text{ g}} = \frac{60\text{ mg}}{1\text{ gr}}$$

Cross-multiply the equation, divide both sides by 1 gr, and then cancel like units to isolate X. There are 120 mg in 2 gr. The bottle is labeled 120 mg/ml; therefore, you should administer 1 ml.

20. B. Set up the equation with X as the unknown quantity:

$$\frac{X}{10\text{ U}} = \frac{1\text{ ml}}{100\text{ U}}$$

Cross-multiply both sides of the equation. To isolate X, divide both sides by 100 U. Finish the math.

21. A. Set up the equation using X as the unknown quantity:

$$\frac{X}{20\text{ mEq}} = \frac{15\text{ ml}}{60\text{ mEq}}$$

Cross multiply the fractions. Then find X by dividing both sides by 60 mEq to isolate X and cancel like units. Finish the math.

22. A. To convert 148, break it into its component parts (100, 40, and 8); then translate into Roman numerals.

23. C. In the correct answer, *qd* is interpreted as "every day" and *0900* is the military time for 9 a.m. Also, *mg* stands for milligrams not grams and *P.O.* means "by mouth" or "orally."

24. B. This answer is incomplete because the unit of measure for the dose is missing.

25. C. *SL* is the abbreviation for sublingual, which means "under the tongue."

26. A. Scheduled drugs are considered on time if they're given one-half hour before or after the ordered time.

27. C. When a controlled substance is removed from the locked storage site, the date and time the dose is removed, the patient's full name, the doctor's name, the drug dose, and your signature must be recorded on the perpetual inventory record. You may also be required to note the amount of the controlled substance remaining in the locked storage site.

28. B. Document the time of administration of a drug immediately after giving the drug to the patient to keep from mistakenly giving the drug again.

29. C. Set up the equation with 200 mg equals 1 tablet as the known amount and X as the unknown factor:

$$\frac{200 \text{ mg}}{1 \text{ tablet}} = \frac{X}{2 \text{ tablets}}$$

Solve for X.

30. B. The generic name is the accepted nonproprietary name, which is a simplified form of the drug's chemical name.

31. A. Set up the equation with 2.5 mg equals 1 tablet as the known factor and X as the unknown factor:

$$\frac{2.5 \text{ mg}}{1 \text{ tablet}} = \frac{5 \text{ mg}}{X}$$

Solve for X.

32. C. Set up the equation with 1 tsp equals 15 ml as the known factor and X as the unknown factor:

$$\frac{1 \text{ tsp}}{15 \text{ ml}} = \frac{1.5 \text{ tsp}}{X}$$

Solve for X.

33. C. Set up the equation with 120 mg per 1 supp as the known factor and X as the unknown factor:

$$120 \text{ mg} : 1 \text{ supp} = 240 \text{ mg} : X$$

Solve for X.

34. A. Set up the equation with 5 mg equals 1 supp as the known factor and X as the unknown factor:

$$5 \text{ mg} : 1 \text{ supp} = 2.5 \text{ mg} : X$$

Solve for X.

35. B. Topical preparations may contain one or more ingredients and you need to make sure the patient isn't allergic to any of them.

36. C. A new patch is applied daily (usually in the morning) and removed after 12 to 14 hours to prevent the patient from developing a tolerance to the drug.

37. B. Set up the equation with the known factor 100 mg/1ml and X as the unknown factor:

$$\frac{100 \text{ mg}}{1 \text{ ml}} = \frac{75 \text{ mg}}{X}$$

Solve for X.

38. A. Set up the equation with the known factor 4 mg/1 ml and X as the unknown factor:

$$\frac{4 \text{ mg}}{1 \text{ ml}} = \frac{3 \text{ mg}}{X}$$

Solve for X. Then subtract the answer (0.75 ml) from 1 ml to determine the amount to waste.

39. C. Set up the equation with 20,000 U/1 ml as the known factor and X as the unknown factor:

$$\frac{20{,}000 \text{ U}}{1 \text{ ml}} = \frac{8000 \text{ U}}{X}$$

Solve for X.

40. B. Set up the equation with 100 units/1 ml as the known factor and X as the unknown factor:

$$\frac{100 \text{ U}}{1 \text{ ml}} = \frac{45 \text{ U}}{X}$$

Solve for X. Cross-multiply the fractions. Then find X by dividing both sides by 100 U to isolate X and cancel like units. Finish the math.

41. C. Convert hours to minutes. Then set up the equation using the formula: Total ml/total minutes × drip factor in drops/ml.

$$X = \frac{100 \text{ ml}}{60 \text{ min}} \times \frac{15 \text{ gtt}}{1 \text{ ml}}$$

Multiply the fraction by the drip factor and cancel like units. Solve for X by dividing the numerator by the demoninator.

42. A. Set up the equation using the formula total volume ordered ÷ number of hours.

43. B. Set up the equation using 25,000 U/500 ml as the known factor and X ml as the unknown factor:

$$\frac{25,000 \text{ U}}{500 \text{ ml}} = \frac{750 \text{ U}}{X}$$

Solve for X.

44. A. Divide the weight in pounds by 2.2 kg (1 lb = 2.2 kg), and round off the answer (20.9) to 21.

45. C. Set up the proportion with the ordered dosage in one fraction and the unknown dosage and the patient's weight in the other fraction:

$$\frac{10 \text{ mg}}{1 \text{ kg}} = \frac{X}{6 \text{ kg}}$$

Cross-multiply, cancel like units, and solve for X.

46. B. First, convert the child's weight to kilograms by dividing by 2.2 kg. Then calculate the dosage, remembering that the first 20 kg of a child's weight requires 1,500 ml and each additional 20 kg of weight requires 20 ml/kg. Because the child weighs 30 kg, he needs 1,500 ml for the first 20 kg and 200 ml for the additional 10 kg of weight.

47. B. First determine the concentration of the solution by setting up the equation with 10 U/1,000 ml as the known factor and X as the unknown factor:

$$\frac{10 \text{ U}}{1000 \text{ ml}} = \frac{X}{1 \text{ ml}}$$

Cross-multiply and solve for X. Then convert to mU by multiplying by 1,000. Next, determine the flow rate by setting up the equation with 10 mU/1 ml as the known factor and 15 mU/X as the unknown factor:

$$\frac{10\ \text{mU}}{1\ \text{ml}} = \frac{15\ \text{mU}}{X}$$

Cross-multiply and solve for X. Convert to an hourly rate by multiplying by 4 (60 minutes/15 minutes = 4).

48. C. Using the calculation for the solution above, 10 mU/1 ml, determine that the patient needs 120 mU in 1 hour (2 mU/minute × 60 minutes). Set up the equation with 10 mU/1 ml as the known factor and 120 mU/X as the unknown factor:

$$\frac{10\ \text{mU}}{1} = \frac{120\ \text{mU}}{X}$$

Cross-multiply and solve for X.

49. C. Set up the equation with 4 g/250 ml as the known factor and 1 g/X as the unknown factor:

$$\frac{4\ \text{g}}{250\ \text{ml}} = \frac{1\ \text{g}}{X}$$

Cross-multiply and solve for X. Round off the answer.

50. A. First find the fluid's strength by setting up the equation 150 mg/500 ml as the known factor and X g/1 ml as the unknown factor:

$$\frac{150\ \text{mg}}{500\ \text{ml}} = \frac{X}{1\ \text{ml}}$$

Cross-multiply and solve for X to determine 0.3 mg/ml of magnesium sulfate. Next, set up the equation with 1 ml/0.3 mg as the known factor and X/0.15 mg as the unknown factor:

$$\frac{1\ \text{ml}}{0.5\ \text{mg}} = \frac{X}{0.15\ \text{mg}}$$

Cross-multiply and solve for X.

51. A. First determine the patient's weight in kilograms by dividing his weight in pounds by 2.2 kg (170 ÷ 2.2 = 77 kg).

Next, determine the concentration of medication in micrograms by multiplying milligrams by 1,000. Then divide by 500 ml to determine the concentration in 1 ml.

$$\frac{800 \text{ mg}}{500 \text{ ml}} \times \frac{1,000 \text{ mcg}}{1 \text{ mg}} = \frac{800,000 \text{ mcg}}{500 \text{ ml}} = \frac{1,600 \text{ mcg}}{1 \text{ ml}}$$

To find out how many milliliters per hour you should give, use the formula: weight in kg $\times$ dose in mcg/kg/min $\times$ 60 (minutes in 1 hour) ÷ concentration in 1 ml of solution:

$$\frac{77 \text{ kg}}{1} \times \frac{5 \text{ mcg}}{\text{kg/min}} = \frac{385 \text{ mcg}}{1 \text{ min}}$$

$$\frac{385 \text{ mcg}}{\text{min}} \times \frac{60 \text{ min}}{1 \text{ hr}} = \frac{23,100 \text{ mcg}}{1 \text{ hr}}$$

$$\frac{23,100 \text{ mcg/hr}}{1,600 \text{ mcg/ml}} = 14.43 \text{ ml/hr}$$

Then round off the answer.

52. C. First, determine the concentration. It's easier to do this if you first convert the 25 mg of nitroglycerin to micrograms by multiplying by 1,000. Then divide this by the number of milliliters to determine the concentration of the solution. Then determine ml/hour by multiplying the ordered dose by 60 minutes and dividing by the concentration.

53. B. Multiply 1 g by 1,000 to convert to milligrams. Then set up the equation with 1,000 mg/250 ml as the known factor and X as the unknown factor to determine the concentration in 1 ml:

$$\frac{1000 \text{ mg}}{250 \text{ ml}} = \frac{X}{1 \text{ ml}}$$

Cross-multiply and solve for X. Using this information, set up an equation with the concentration per milliliter as the known factor and 3 mg/X as the unknown factor:

$$\frac{4 \text{ mg}}{1 \text{ ml}} = \frac{3 \text{ mg}}{X}$$

Cross-multiply and solve for X. You find 0.75 ml for 3 mg of lidocaine. Now set up the final equation with 0.75 ml/1 minute and X/60 minutes. Cross-multiply and solve for X.

Glossary

Apothecaries' system: system used to measure liquid volumes and solid weights based on the units *drop, minim,* and *grain,* with amounts expressed in Roman numerals; used before the metric system was established

Avoirdupois system: measurement system used to order certain pharmaceutical products and to weigh patients; based on the units *grain, ounce,* and *pound*

body surface area (BSA): the area covered by a person's external skin calculated in square meters (m²) according to height and weight; used to calculate safe pediatric dosages for all drugs and safe dosages for adult patients receiving extremely potent drugs or drugs requiring great precision, such as antineoplastic and chemotherapeutic agents

common factor: a number that's a factor of two different numbers (For example, 2 is a common factor of 4 and 6.)

common fraction: fraction with a whole number in both the numerator and denominator (such as ⅔)

complex fraction: fraction in which the numerator and denominator also are fractions such as:

$$\frac{2/7}{5/16}$$

concentration: ratio that expresses the amount of a drug in a solution; sometimes called drug strength

denominator: the bottom number in a fraction, which represents the total number of equal parts of a whole (For example, in the fraction ⁷⁄₁₀, the denominator is 10.)

dividend: in division, the number to be divided (For example, in the problem 33 ÷ 7, 33 is the dividend.)

divisor: in division, the number by which the dividend is divided (For example, in the problem 33 ÷ 7, 7 is the divisor.)

dosage: the amount, frequency, and number of doses of a drug

dose: the amount of a drug to be given at one time

drip factor: the number of drops to be delivered per milliliter of solution in an I.V. administration set; measured in gtt/ml (drops per milliliter); listed on the package containing the I.V. tubing administration set

drip rate: the number of drops of I.V. solution to be infused per minute; based on the drip factor (number of drops delivered per millimeter) and calibrated for the selected I.V. tubing

enteral: within or by way of the small intestine

equianalgesic dose: amount of a narcotic that provides the same pain relief as 10 mg of intramuscular morphine; used to recalculate the necessary dose when substituting one analgesic for another

flow rate: the number of milliliters of I.V. fluid to administer over 1 hour; based on the total volume to be infused in milliliters and the amount of time for the infusion

fraction: representation of the division of one number by another number; mathematical expression for parts of a whole, with the bottom number (denominator) describing the total number of parts and the top number (numerator) describing

the parts of the whole being considered (for example, ½, ⅓, ⁷⁄₁₈)

generic name: accepted nonproprietary name, which is a simplified form of the drug's chemical name

glucometer: device used to calculate blood glucose levels — and, thereby, insulin levels — from a drop of blood

grain: the basic unit for measuring solid weight in the Apothecaries' system

gram (g): basic unit of weight in the metric system; represents the weight of one cubic centimeter of water at 4° C

household system: system that uses familiar household items, such as teaspoons, to measure drugs

improper fraction: fraction in which the numerator is larger than or equal to the denominator, such as ³⁄₂, ¹⁰⁄₇, and ⅝

International System of Units: system adopted in 1960 by the International Bureau of Weights and Measures to promote the use of standard metric abbreviations to prevent drug transcription errors

intradermal route: drug administration into the dermis of the skin

intramuscular route (I.M.): drug administration into a muscle

intravenous route (I.V.): drug administration into a vein

largest common divisor: in a fraction, the largest whole number that can be divided into both the numerator and denominator of a fraction (For example, in the fraction ⁸⁄₁₀, the largest common divisor is 2.)

liter (L): basic unit of fluid volume in the metric system; equivalent to $\frac{1}{10}$ of a cubic meter

lowest common denominator: smallest number that's a multiple of all denominators in a set of fractions; also called least common multiple (For example, for the fractions, $\frac{1}{100}$ and $\frac{3}{150}$, the lowest common denominator is 300.)

lowest terms: in a fraction, the smallest numbers possible in the numerator and denominator (Reduce a fraction to its lowest terms by dividing the numerator and denominator by the largest common divisor. For example, in the fraction $\frac{3}{15}$, divide both the numerator and denominator by 3, the largest common divisor, to find $\frac{1}{5}$, the lowest terms of this fraction.)

meter (m): basic unit of length in the metric system; equivalent to 39.37 inches

metric system: decimal-based measurement system that uses the units *meter* (for length), *liter* (for volume), and *gram* (for weight); most widely used system for measuring amounts of drugs

milliequivalent (mEq): number of grams of a solute in 1 ml of normal solution; used to measure electrolytes

minim: basic unit for measuring liquid volume in the Apothecaries' system

mixed number: number that consists of a whole number and a fraction (such as $1\frac{1}{2}$)

multiplied common denominator: for a set of fractions, the product of all the denominators, which is found by multiplying all the denominators together (For example, for the fractions, $\frac{1}{2}$, $\frac{2}{3}$, and $\frac{3}{5}$, multiply the denominators together to find the multiplied common denominator, which is 30 [$2 \times 3 \times 5 = 30$].)

nonparenteral drugs: drugs administered by the oral, topical, or rectal route, as opposed to drugs administered by the parenteral route

nomogram: chart used to determine body surface area in square meters, based on the patient's height and weight

numerator: the top number in a fraction, which represents the number of parts being considered (For example, in the fraction $\frac{7}{10}$, the numerator is 7.)

oral route (P.O.): drug administration through the mouth

parenteral route: drug administration through a route other than the digestive tract, such as I.V., intramuscularly, and subcutaneously

percentage: a quantity stated as a part per hundred; written with a percent sign (%), which means "for every hundred" (For example, 50% represents 50 parts out of 100 total parts.)

prime factor: prime numbers that can be divided into some part of a mathematical expression such as the denominators in a set of fractions; used to find the lowest common denominator for a set of fractions (For example, the prime factors for the denominators in the fractions $\frac{1}{10}$ and $\frac{2}{3}$ are 5, 2, and 3.)

prime number: whole number that's evenly divisible only by 1 and itself, such as 2, 3, 5, and 7

product: the answer of a multiplication problem (For example, in the equation, $4 \times 5 = 20$, the product is 20.)

proper fraction: fraction with a numerator that's smaller than the denominator (such as $\frac{1}{2}$)

proportion: set of equivalent ratios or fractions (An example of a proportion expressed by ratios is 2 : 3 :: 8 : 12, which is read as "2 is to 3 as 8 is to 12." The same proportion expressed with fractions is $\frac{2}{3} = \frac{8}{12}$.)

quotient: the answer of a division problem (For example, in the equation $20 \div 5 = 4$, the quotient is 4.)

ratio: numerical way to compare items or show a relationship between numbers, with numbers separated by a colon, which represents the words, "is to" (For example, the ratio 4 : 5 is read as "4 is to 5." Ratios are commonly used to describe the relative proportions of ingredients such as the amount of drug relative to its solution.)

reciprocal: inverted fraction; used when dividing fractions (For example, to divide $\frac{1}{2}$ by $\frac{2}{3}$, multiply $\frac{1}{2}$ by the reciprocal of $\frac{2}{3}$, which is $\frac{3}{2}$; in other words, $\frac{1}{2} \div \frac{2}{3} = \frac{1}{2} \times \frac{3}{2} = \frac{3}{4}$. When a fraction is multiplied by its reciprocal, the product is 1; for example, the reciprocal of the fraction $\frac{2}{3}$ is $\frac{3}{2}$, and $\frac{2}{3} \times \frac{3}{2} = \frac{6}{6}$ or 1.)

rectal route (P.R.): drug administration (usually by suppository) through the rectum

reduce: to simplify a numerical expression by using the lowest possible numbers — or lowest terms — to describe it (For example, the fraction $\frac{15}{45}$ may be reduced to $\frac{1}{3}$.)

rounding off: reducing the number of decimal places used to express a number (For example, a decimal fraction that's expressed in thousandths may be rounded off to the nearest hundredths or tenths; the number 12.827 rounded off to the nearest hundredths is 12.83. The same number rounded off to the nearest tenths is 12.8.)

subcutaneous route (S.C.): drug administration into the subcutaneous tissue

topical route: drug administration through the skin (after absorption through the skin layers, the drug enters circulation), usually in cream, ointment, or transdermal patch form

trade name: the drug's name given by the manufacturer; also called the brand or proprietary name

transcribe: to write or type a copy of something; to record information by hand, tape-recorder, or computer

transdermal route: drug administration in which the drug is absorbed continuously through the skin and enters the systemic system

unit system: measurement system that expresses the amount of a drug in units (U), United States Pharmacopeia (USP) units, or International Units (IU) (Drugs measured in units include insulin, heparin, the topical antibiotic bacitracin, and penicillins G and V. Some forms of vitamins A and D are measured in USP units. The hormone calcitonin and the fat-soluble vitamins A, D, and E are measured in IUs.)

Index

A

Abbreviations
  approved, in drug orders, 110, 111-112t
  use of, in metric system, 77, 78, 79
Acetaminophen, calculating dosage of, 146-147, 158, 168
Additives for I.V. infusions, 226-228
Adenosine, calculating dosage for, 271-272
Administration records, 121-130
  avoiding transcription errors on, 128-130
  documentation on, 124-128
  types of systems used for, 121-123, 123i
Administration schedule, recording, on administration record, 126
Amoxicillin, calculating dosage of, 239-240
Ampicillin, calculating dosage of, 201-202
Apothecaries' system, 92-94
  conversions in, 92, 93t, 94
  liquid and solid equivalents in, 98t
  Roman numerals in, 92-94
  units of measure in, 92
  uses for, 92
Aspirin, calculating dosage of, 153-154
Avoirdupois system, 97
  solid equivalents in, 98t

B

Blood products, transfusing, 228-229
Blood transfusions, 228-229
Body surface area
  dosage calculation by, 242, 243, 243i
  pediatric fluid needs calculation by, 253
Brethine, 257, 259t

C

Calculator, fraction conversion and, 37i
Calories as basis for calculating pediatric fluid needs, 252-253
Capsule, altering dose of, 146
Carpuject syringe. See Prefilled syringes.
Ceclor, calculating dosage of, 149-150
Centiliters, converting, to liters, 84
Chemotherapy, determining safe dose of, for pediatric patient, 244
Chloral hydrate, calculating dosage of, 244-245
Clonidine transdermal patch, 166
Closed-system prefilled devices, 181
Clozapine, calculating dosage of, 148
Common fraction, 4
  converting, to decimal fraction, 32
  converting, to percentages, 37-38
  converting decimal fraction to, 33-34
  converting percentages to, 35-37
Common-fraction equations, finding value of X in, 48-51
Complex fraction, 4
Computerized record systems, 122
Controlled substances, documenting administration of, 127
Critical care drugs
  calculating I.V. flow rates for, 273-278, 277i
  I.V. injection of, 269-272, 271i
  special considerations for, 278-280
Cross products, 57-58, 57i

D

Dates, recording, on administration record, 125
Decimal fractions, 26
  adding and subtracting, 28-29
  converting, to common fractions, 33-34
  converting, to mixed number, 34-35
  converting common fractions to, 32
  converting mixed numbers to, 32-33
  dividing, 29-30, 31i
  multiplying, 29
  rounding off, 30-32
Decimal-fraction equations, finding value of X in, 52-54
Decimal number, 26
  deleting zeros in, 27, 27i, 28
Decimal point, 26-27, 26i
  in drug orders, 28, 193, 194
  placement of, 28, 29, 30, 35, 36, 81-82, 82i
Decimals, 26-35
  converting percentages to, 35
Denominator, 3i, 4, 14i
  finding common, 8-16
Desired-over-have method, 156-159
Diabetes, types of, 188
Digoxin, calculating dosage of, 155-156, 272
Dilatin, calculating dosage of, 151
Dimensional analysis, 65-73
  conversion factors and, 66
  given quantity and, 66
  setting up problem for, 67
  unwanted units and, 67
  wanted quantity and, 66
Divided doses, 145, 146
Dobutamine, calculating dosage of, 276-278, 277i
Documentation
  controlled substances and, 127
  on administration record, 124-128

i refers to an illustration; t refers to a table.

Dosage calculation
   by body surface area, 242, 243i, 244
   dimensional analysis and, 65-73
   for critical care drugs, 273-278, 277i
   for I.V. push, 270-272
   for obstetric patient, 260-266, 261i
   for oral drugs, 135-159
   for pediatric patient, 235-253
   in milligrams per kilogram of body
      weight, 238-241
Dosage form, recording, on administration record, 125
Dose strength, drug label and, 137i,
   138-139
Drip factor, 207
Drip rates, calculating, 207-210, 208t,
   211-212
Dropper, checking fluid measurement
   in, 95i
Drug errors
   preventing, 128-130, 137i
   reporting, 130
Drug information, recording, on administration record, 124-128
Drug label
   for critical care drugs, 270, 271i,
      277i
   for obstetric drugs, 260, 261i
   for oral drugs, 135-139, 136i, 137,
      138i
   for parenteral drugs, 185-188, 186i,
      186t, 187t
   for rectal drugs, 163, 164i, 165
   for topical drugs, 163, 164i, 165
   interpreting percentage solution on,
      186, 186t, 187
   interpreting ratio solutions on, 186,
      187-188, 187t
Drug name
   on drug label, 135-137, 136i, 137i
   recording, on administration
      record, 125

Drug orders, 109-118
   approved abbreviations for, 110,
      111-112t
   clarifying information on, 114, 116,
      117i, 118
   components of, 110
   converting, to equivalent measure-
      ments, 102-104
   decimal point in, 28, 193, 194
   discontinuing, 115
   drug administration timing and, 114
   for insulin, 191-193, 194
   guidelines for writing, 110
   interpreting, 115t, 116
   methods of generating, 109-110
   military time requirement for,
      113-114, 113i
   refusing to carry out, 129
   renewing, 114
   transcription of, to administration
      record, 124-126, 127-128
Drug strength, recording, on administration record, 125
Dulcolax, calculating dosage of,
   168-169

E

Electrolyte infusions, 226
Electronic infusion devices, 216-218
Ephedrine, calculating dosage of, 242,
   244
Equianalgesic charts, 145, 147t
Equivalent measure conversions,
   103-104
Erythromycin, calculating dosage of,
   150-151
Estradiol transdermal patch, 166
Expiration date, drug label and, 139

F

Factor analysis. *See* Dimensional
   analysis.
Factor labeling. *See* Dimensional
   analysis.

Fentanyl transdermal system, 165, 166
Fetal assessment, obstetric drug administration and, 256, 257
Filter needles, 182i
Five rights of drug administration, 118
Fluid needs of pediatric patient, calculating, 250-253
   based on body surface area, 253
   based on calories, 252-253
   based on weight, 250-252
Fractions, 3-22
   adding, 16-18, 17i
   as parts of whole, 3-4, 3i
   changing whole numbers to, 50, 51i
   comparing relative size of, 13-16
   converting, to mixed numbers, 6
   converting, to same denominator,
      10-13
   converting mixed numbers to, 5-6
   dividing, 21-22
   finding common denominator for,
      8-16
   multiplying, 20-21
   numerical relationships and, 45, 46
   reducing, to lowest terms, 7
   subtracting, 17i, 18-20
   types of, 4
   using, in proportions, 47-48, 57-59

G

Gentamicin, calculating dosage of,
   200-201
Glyburide, calculating dosage of,
   148-149
Gram, 77
   converting, to milligram, 83

H

Heparin
   calculating dosage of, 99, 100,
      194-195
   calculating flow rate for, 221-223
   calculating units per hour, 223-224
   dosage calculation errors with, 195

i refers to an illustration; t refers to a table.

Hetastarch, calculating infusion time for, 214-215
Hollow-handle spoon, checking fluid measurement in, 95i
Household system, 95-97
    conversions in, 95-97
    liquid equivalents in, 98t
    units of measure in, 95, 96
    uses for, 95

IJ

I.M. injections, 177. *See also* Parenteral injection.
    administering, to pediatric patient, 237-238, 237i
I.M. needles, 182i
Improper fraction, 4
    converting, to mixed number, 6
    converting mixed numbers to, 5-6
Insulin, 188
    action times for, 192t
    calculating continuous infusion of, 224-225
    calculating dosage of, 195
    combining, in same syringe, 193-194
    concentrations of, 190
    initials for, 189
    origins of, 188-189
    reading labels on, 189, 190i
    reading orders for, 191-193, 194
    sliding scale for, 192-193, 196, 196t
    subtypes of, 191t
    types of, 188-190
    unit label on, 188, 189i
    unit measurement of, 99
International System of Units, 80
Intradermal injections, 176. *See also* Parenteral injection.
Intradermal needles, 182i
I.V. bag
    as information source, 206i
    time-taping, 217i

I.V. infusion
    adjusting rate of, 220
    administering additives by, 226-228
    administering blood and blood products by, 228-229
    administering total parenteral nutrition by, 229-230
    assessing, 206
    calculating continuous insulin administration by, 224-225
    calculating drip rates for, 207-210, 208t, 211-212
    calculating flow rate for, 210
    calculating piggyback dose for, 227
    calculating time required for, 212-215
    continuous, 248
    critical care drugs and, 269-272, 271i
    intermittent, 248-249, 248i
    regulating, 216-220, 219i
    selecting tubing for, 206-207
    time-taping bag for, 217i
    volume-control devices and, 248-249, 249i
I.V. injection, administering, to pediatric patient, 238, 248-249, 249i
I.V. needles, 182i
I.V. pumps
    advantages of, 216-217
    regulating I.V. flow with, 217-218
I.V. push, 269
    calculating dosages for, 270-272

K

Kardex medication record system, 121, 123i
Kilometer, converting meter to, 81-83

L

Lactated Ringer's solution, calculating infusion time for, 215
Lidocaine, calculating dosage of, 274-276

Liter, 77
    converting centiliters to, 84

M

Macrodrip tubing, 207
Magnesium sulfate, 257, 259t, 260
    calculating dosage of, 263-264
Manual regulation of I.V. flow, 216
Maternal assessment, obstetric drug administration and, 255-256, 257
Measurement system
    apothecaries', 92-94
    avoirdupois, 97
    household, 95-97
    milliequivalent, 100-102
    metric, 77-88
    selecting, 91
    unit, 98-100
Medication administration record system, 122
Medication cup, checking fluid measurement in, 95i
Meter, 77
    converting, to kilometer, 81-83
Metric conversions, 80-84, 81t
    decimal placement in, 81-82, 82i, 83, 84
    finding value of X in, 84-87
Metric graduate, 79i
Metric mathematics, 87-88
Metric ruler, 79i
Metric system, 77-88
    abbreviations used in, 77, 78, 79
    advantages of, 77
    liquid and solid equivalents in, 98t
    measuring devices used with, 79i
    prefixes in, 78-79, 80t
    tips when using, 78t
    units of measurement in, 77-78, 79
Metric weights, 79i
Microdrip tubing, 207

i refers to an illustration; t refers to a table.

Milliequivalent system, 100-102
    conversions in, 101-102
    electrolyte measurement in, 100,
        101
    uses for, 100-101
Milligram, converting gram to, 83
Mixed number
    converting, to decimal fractions,
        32-33
    converting, to improper fraction, 5-6
    converting decimal fractions to,
        34-35
    converting improper fraction to, 6

N

Needles, types of, 182, 182i
Nicotine transdermal patch, 166
Nitroglycerin transdermal patch, 166
Nitroprusside, calculating dosage of,
        279
Nomogram, dosage calculation and,
        243i
Normal saline solution, calculating
        infusion time for, 213-214
Numerator, 3i, 4
Numerical relationships, 45-48
Nutrient infusions, 226

O

Obstetric drug administration, 255
    dosage calculation and, 260-266,
        261i
    drugs used in, 256-257, 258-259t, 260
    fetal assessment and, 256, 257
    maternal assessment and, 255-256,
        257
Ointment, measuring dose of, 166-167,
        167i

Oral drugs, 135
    administering, to pediatric patient,
        236-237, 238
    calculating dosages of, 141-145
    converting dosage of, to equivalent
        measure, 152-159
    in liquid form, 149-152
    in solid form, 144-145, 146
    reading labels on, 135-139, 136i,
        137i, 138i
    safe administration of, 139-141
    special considerations for, 145-146,
        147t
Oral solutions, measuring, 152
Oxytocin, 258t, 260
    calculating dosage of, 260-263

PQ

Package insert as information source,
        198i
Parenteral injection, 175
    interpreting drug label for, 185-188,
        185i, 186t, 187t
    recording site of, on administration
        record, 126
    types of, 175-176
Patient-controlled analgesia pump,
        218-220, 219i
    benefits of, 218
    checking accuracy of, 220
    preparation guidelines for, 218-219
    recording drug dosage with,
        219-220
    safety features of, 218
Patient information, recording, on
        administration record, 124
PCA. *See* Patient-controlled analgesia
        pump.
Pediatric dosages
    factors that influence, 235
    methods for calculating, 238-244,
        243i
    verifying, 244-247

Pediatric patient
    administering drugs to, 236-238
    calculating fluid needs of, 250-253
    I.V. guidelines for, 248-249, 248i
Penicillin, calculating dosage of,
        99-100, 199-200, 240-241, 245-247
Percentage problems, solving, 38-43
Percentages, 35-38
    converting, to common fractions,
        35-37
    converting, to decimals, 35
    converting common fractions to,
        37-38
Percentage solutions, interpreting,
        186, 186t, 187
Percent sign, 35
Phenobarbital, calculating dosage of,
        154-155, 158-159
Phenylephrine in saline solution, cal-
        culating dosage of, 279-278
Pitocin, 258t, 260
Potassium chloride
    calculating I.V. dosage of, 101
    calculating oral dosage of, 102, 157
Powders
    diluting, 151-152
    in two-chamber vials, 197, 198i
    multiple-strength, 196
    reconstituting, 196-202, 198t, 198i,
        199i
    single-strength, 196
Prefilled syringes, 179-181, 181i
Prime factor, 8
Prime factoring, 8-9
Prime number, 8
Procainamide, calculating dosage for,
        270-271, 271i
Proper fraction, 4
Proportions
    numerical relationships and, 45
    using fractions in, 47-48, 57-59, 143
    using ratios in, 46-47, 54-57, 142, 143

R

Ratios
  numerical relationships and, 45, 46
  using, in proportions, 46-47, 54-57
Ratio solutions, interpreting, 187-188,
    187t
Reconstituting powders, 196-202, 198t,
    199i
Record-keeping systems for drug
    administration, 121-123, 123i
Rectal drugs, 163
  calculating dosages of, 167-169
  reading labels on, 163, 164i, 165
Refusal to administer drug, 129
Roman numerals, apothecaries' sys-
    tem and, 92-94
Route of administration, recording, on
    administration record, 126

S

S.C. injection. *See* Subcutaneous
    injections.
Scopolamine transdermal patch, 166
Signature on administration record,
    127-128
Sodium bicarbonate, calculating
    dosage of, 101-102
Solute, 186
Solution, 186
Special delivery drug dosages, 142
Special orders, recording, on adminis-
    tration record, 126
Subcutaneous injections, 176-177. *See
    also* Parenteral injection.
  administering, to pediatric patient,
    237, 238
Subcutaneous needles, 182i
Suppository
  calculating dosage for, 167-169
  reading label on, 164i

Syringes
  calibration marks on, 178-179
  components of, 178i, 180i, 181i
  insulin, 190, 193i
  types of, 178-182

T

Tablet, altering dose of, 145, 146
Terbutaline, 257, 259t
  calculating dosage of, 264-266
Testosterone transdermal patch, 166
Thiamine, calculating dosage and flow
    rate for, 226-228
Tigan, calculating dosage of, 169
Time of administration, recording, on
    administration record, 127
Topical drugs, 163
  calculating dosages of, 166-167
  measuring, 167i
  reading labels on, 163, 164i, 165
  transdermal patches and, 165-166
Total parenteral nutrition, administer-
    ing, 229-230
Transdermal patches, 165-166
  absorption of, 165
  disadvantages of, 165
  drugs used in, 165-166
  rate of release and, 165
Tuberculin syringes, 179, 180i
Tubex syringe. *See* Prefilled syringes.

U

Unit-dose packaging, 141, 141i
Unit system, 98-100
  conversions in, 99-100
  drugs measured in, 98-99

V

Verifying pediatric dosages, 244-247
Volume-control devices, 248-249, 248i

Volume per volume solution, determin-
    ing contents of, 186t, 187, 187t

W

Weight as basis for calculating pedi-
    atric fluid needs, 250-252
Weight per volume solution, determin-
    ing contents of, 186t, 187, 187t
Whole numbers, changing, into frac-
    tions, 50, 51i

XYZ

X, finding value of, 48-63
  in common-fraction equations,
    48-51
  in decimal-fraction equations, 52-54
  in dosage calculations, 49
  in proportion problems with frac-
    tions, 57-59
  in proportion problems with ratios,
    54-57
  metric unit conversion and, 84-87

Notes

Notes

Notes

Notes

Notes